D0984709

TREATING DEPRESSED
AND SUICIDAL ADOLESCENTS

TREATING DEPRESSED AND SUICIDAL ADOLESCENTS

A CLINICIAN'S GUIDE

David A. Brent
Kimberly D. Poling
Tina R. Goldstein

THE GUILFORD PRESS
New York   London

© 2011 The Guilford Press
A Division of Guilford Publications, Inc.
72 Spring Street, New York, NY 10012
www.guilford.com

Printed in the United States of America

This book is printed on acid-free paper.

Last digit is print number: 9 8 7 6 5 4 3 2 1

The authors have checked with sources believed to be reliable in their efforts to provide information that is complete and generally in accord with the standards of practice that are accepted
at the time of publication. However, in view of the possibility of human error or changes in
medical sciences, neither the authors, nor the editor and publisher, nor any other party who
has been involved in the preparation or publication of this work warrants that the information
contained herein is in every respect accurate or complete, and they are not responsible for
any errors or omissions or the results obtained from the use of such information. Readers are
encouraged to confirm the information contained in this book with other sources.

Library of Congress Cataloging-in-Publication Data

Brent, David A.
  Treating depressed and suicidal adolescents: a clinician's guide / David A. Brent,
Kimberly D. Poling, and Tina R. Goldstein.
     p. ; cm.
  Includes bibliographical references and index.
  ISBN 978-1-60623-957-5 (hardcover: alk. paper)
  1. Depression in adolescence—Treatment.   2. Adolescent psychotherapy.
3. Teenagers—Suicidal behavior.   I. Poling, Kimberly D.   II. Goldstein, Tina R.
III. Title.
  [DNLM: 1. Depressive Disorder—psychology.   2. Depressive Disorder—
therapy.   3. Adolescent Behavior—psychology.   4. Adolescent Psychology.
5. Suicide—prevention & control.   6. Suicide—psychology.   WM 171]
  RJ506.D4B74 2011
  616.85′2700835—dc22
                                                                    2010028727

Whoever destroys a single life,
it is as if he destroyed an entire world.
And whoever saves a single life,
it is as if he saved an entire world,
because each person is a unique creation.
Therefore every single person is obligated to say,
"The world was created for me."
(Paraphrased from *Mishna Sanhedrin* 4:5)

About the Authors

David A. Brent, MD, is Academic Chief of Child and Adolescent Psychiatry at the University of Pittsburgh School of Medicine and holds an Endowed Chair in Suicide Studies. He is Director of Services for Teens at Risk (STAR-Center), a clinical service for depressed and suicidal teens. Dr. Brent has conducted some of the most important work on the risk factors for depression and suicidal behavior in adolescents, and has successfully translated that work into the development and testing of effective pharmacological and psychotherapeutic interventions for depressed and suicidal adolescents. He has received wide recognition for his contributions on the assessment and treatment of depressed and suicidal adolescents, including research awards from the American Foundation for Suicide Prevention, the American Association of Suicidology, the National Alliance for Research on Schizophrenia and Depression, the American Academy of Child and Adolescent Psychiatry, and the American Psychiatric Association.

Kimberly D. Poling, LCSW, is Clinical Program Manager at the STAR-Center, which she initially joined as a therapist in 1987. She has been involved in developing and implementing treatment protocols, training, and supervising cognitive therapists, both in Pittsburgh and throughout the country, and is an expert in the areas of cognitive therapy, diagnostic assessment, and suicide risk assessment. She has also served as a faculty member at the Center for Cognitive Therapy at the University of Pittsburgh Medical Center and in the Department of Psychology and Education of the University of Pittsburgh.

Tina R. Goldstein, PhD, a clinical psychologist, is Assistant Professor in the Department of Child and Adolescent Psychiatry at the University of Pittsburgh School of Medicine. Her clinical and research interests focus on the development and testing of psychosocial interventions for children and adolescents with and at risk for mood disorders, as well as the prevention and treatment of suicidal behavior in youth. Dr. Goldstein is the recipient of multiple foundation and federal grants for which she conducts, trains, and supervises psychosocial treatment protocols for youth. She has expertise in cognitive-behavioral therapy and dialectical behavior therapy.

Acknowledgments

We gratefully acknowledge all those who have had a critical role in helping us find our way.

First, we are indebted to Dr. Aaron Beck, the founder of cognitive-behavioral therapy (CBT), for providing the foundation for the treatment we have developed. Dr. Robert Berchick and, more recently, Dr. Greg Brown have further helped hone our thinking on the application of CBT for suicidal teens.

We appreciate the commitment of all of the Services for Teens At Risk (STAR-Center) faculty and staff, too numerous to list. Several core clinicians at the STAR-Center provided critical contributions to the development of the treatment approach we describe herein:

Boris Birmaher, MD
Charles Bonner, PhD
Mary Beth Boylan, PhD
Maureen Maher-Bridge, LCSW
Charles Goldstein, LCSW
Mary Margaret Kerr, EdD
Brian McKain, MSN
Grace Moritz, LCSW
Mary Wartella, LCSW
Susan Wesner, MSN

We would like to acknowledge the Treatment of Adolescent Suicide Attempters (TASA) research team, particularly Barbara Stanley, PhD, Karen Wells, PhD, Betsy Kennard, PsyD, and John Curry, PhD. As we articulated the treatment principles we developed in our clinic over many years to these expert clinicians and researchers, they helped us to refine its presentation, and to realize that we had something of great value to share.

We are grateful to the following agencies for supporting our work: the Commonwealth of Pennsylvania, the National Institute of Mental Health, the American Foundation for Suicide Prevention, the W. T. Grant Foundation, and the National Alliance for Research on Schizophrenia and Depression.

We dedicate this book to our past, present, and future STAR-Center patients and their families.

Finally, we would like to thank our families, who have supported us and kept us grounded so that we could meet the challenges of treating depressed and suicidal adolescents.

Please note: All names and identifying information in the case examples we describe are fictional. These case examples are not based on any one individual patient or family member. In order to include realistic clinical examples, we have drawn from clinical material amassed from a multitude of patients we have seen at the STAR-Center over the years.

Contents

xi

Introduction

One might ask, why write a book about adolescents who are both depressed and suicidal? The simple answer is that these patients are all-too-common visitors to the emergency room and hospital and are a major challenge to the clinician. Common as these patients are, there is not much in the literature to guide the clinician, because they are often excluded from clinical trials. Thus, much of the extant data about teen depression does not necessarily inform us about how to care for these patients. Yet suicidal thoughts and behavior are very common in patients with depression, so the ability to assess and treat patients with these interrelated conditions is an important component in the care of young patients with mood disorders. Moreover, while suicidal ideation and behavior are associated with greater severity and chronicity of depression, it is clear that there are many depressed individuals who never become suicidal. Thus there must be, and indeed there are, factors above and beyond depression that contribute to suicidality and require distinct interventions. The focus on both of these vulnerabilities simultaneously is unique and, we argue, necessary to properly care for these high-risk youth. This preface records some of the key events along the way that have shaped our approach to taking care of depressed and suicidal youth.

In 1982, I (D. A. B.) was offered a faculty position at the University of Pittsburgh by Dr. Thomas Detre, one of the most charismatic and visionary medical leaders of the past half century. He was part of an elite group that insisted that psychiatry rejoin the rest of medicine through

1

hard-nosed empiricism. While I was convinced of the importance of empiricism, I was also struck by the impressive results achieved by highly skilled psychoanalytic supervisors and colleagues—in the absence of "empiricism." Clearly they brought to their work something of inordinate value, albeit somewhat intangible and difficult to define. Ironically, this hard-to-define quality was also something Dr. Detre demonstrated in abundance in his astute interviews with patients and in his ability to recruit and develop talented faculty. I started to question what this was: An individual characteristic? A talent one can develop? So, as I was accepting the invitation to join the ranks of the empiricists, I asked Dr. Detre, somewhat wistfully, "But don't you also believe that there is something else, something artful, that does not go out of date?" He laughed and replied, "Yes, but you still need to define and prove it."

This book is a response to the challenge posed to me by Dr. Detre over two decades ago: to combine that which is current and data-based with that which is timeless in order to get the best results for our patients. Best practice must be guided by empirical data. But good clinical care also involves art—the art of establishing a collaborative relationship with the patient in order to jointly make clinical decisions. The therapeutic gains occur at the interface between empiricism and collaboration—*collaborative empiricism,* as it was termed by Dr. Aaron Beck, one of the true creative giants of modern psychiatry and the developer of cognitive therapy. The application of collaborative empiricism to the care of depressed, suicidal adolescents is the primary focus of this book. Although new data will emerge to alter our concept of best practice, it is our hope that the approach described in this book will stand the test of time.

Dr. Thomas Detre came to the Western Psychiatric Institute and Clinic (WPIC) in 1973 and established a culture in which questioning and research could flourish. Always the penultimate judge of talent, Dr. Detre recruited Dr. David Kupfer, who became Chair of the Department of Psychiatry from 1983–2009. This appointment was perhaps most instrumental to the success of WPIC. Dr. Kupfer has arguably done more than any other single individual to advance the treatment of mood disorders, and created a template for the conduct of clinical research that many of us emulate. The late Dr. Joaquim ("Kim") Puig-Antich was among the first of a new breed of empirically oriented child psychiatrists, and encouraged those of us who were slightly younger to take risks and have fun doing it. Dr. Maria Kovacs, who continues to conduct groundbreaking work in pediatric mood disorders, served as my mentor and had the patience to teach me to express my thoughts with a minimum of ambiguity. In my opinion, the most creative American psychiatrist is Dr. Aaron Beck, who has contributed monumentally to both the understanding and treatment of the complex phenomena of depression and suicidality.

These great scientific leaders share a common trait: they were not afraid of failure—in fact, they flourished on it. They delighted in trying to understand why a treatment did not work, or when a theory did not fit. There is a quotation from the Sayings of the Fathers: "I have learned much from my teachers, but more from my students." Through my own experience, I realized I could learn the most from my patients, especially those whom I failed to help, and turn present failure into future success.

Another more personal challenge led me to write this book. In 1979, my brother James died suddenly at the age of 26 of a cardiac arrhythmia. Four months before, we had what turned out to be our last conversation. He was a musician and composer, and I asked him who he was listening to of late. His response was "me." I thought that was incredibly egotistical and told him so. "You don't understand," he said. "The music I want to hear hasn't been written yet, and I'm going to write it." I responded, "You know, the child psychiatry I want to read hasn't been written yet, either. Maybe I'll write some of it, too."

It is important to acknowledge those unseen authors who have shaped this work. I cannot ever thank my parents, Robert and Lillian Brent, adequately for all that they have done for me. They hold as an ideal the life of the mind harnessed to the service of humankind. While my parents provided the genetics, my wife, Nancy, has provided the environment for me to succeed. Having found a soul mate makes everything possible.

My journey in the study of adolescent depression and suicide began around 1980. I was assigned to the consultation–liaison service at Children's Hospital of Pittsburgh and was evaluating approximately three adolescent suicide attempters per week. My main task was to determine whom it was safe to send home and who had to be referred for inpatient services due to high risk for a repeat attempt. One day, I had to determine the disposition for two such patients. I recommended discharge for one and inpatient psychiatric services for the other. The father of the child whom I had referred to the hospital confronted me, wanting to know how I had made my decision; I was not able to explain. I realized that I was close to finishing my training, and I did not even know how to decide who was at risk for suicide. I went to the library to read up on adolescent suicide and was shocked to discover that there was almost nothing written on the subject. I had found the music that I wanted to hear, and realized it had not yet been written.

At that time, our approach to adolescent suicide was comprised of equal parts ignorance and fear. The suicide rate was increasing rapidly, having tripled in previous 20 years. It was commonly believed that a teen who attempted or completed suicide was simply under too much stress and/or misunderstood by his or her parents. An additional misconception was that teen suicide was *not* associated with psychiatric illness. We had very little knowledge about risk factors for suicide or suicidal behavior. There was a great deal of concern about suicide contagion—would one suicide in a high school set off an epidemic? Finally, there were no empirically validated treatments for depression *or* suicidal behavior in adolescents, so that even if we could identify the kids at risk for suicide, we had no idea what to do with them.

In order to determine risk for suicide, it was necessary to know more about adolescents who had completed suicide and compare them to other groups. The central problem with the study of suicide is that people who complete suicide take this vital information with them. Still, there was an approach that had been used in several adult studies, called a psychological autopsy, in which the family and other close contacts are interviewed to reconstruct factors leading up to the suicide. I obtained some funding and began to contact the families of adolescent suicide victims, with great trepidation, in order to talk with them and learn more about what might have gone wrong.

As it turned out, my main problem was not getting in the door of the homes of suicide victims—it was leaving. The families so needed to make some sense out of what happened, and felt so isolated because no one wanted to talk with them about the suicide, that they welcomed the opportunity to go over the factors that led up to the suicide. It became apparent that they had been engaged in this process in their own minds almost incessantly since the tragic event.

We learned that these adolescent suicide completers were not just misunderstood kids. Over 90% of them, by the report of parents, siblings, and friends, had at least one major psychiatric disorder. On average, their psychiatric conditions started 7 years before the suicide. Depression was the single most common psychiatric problem, but it often occurred in combination with other problems, like substance abuse. The depression was usually "normalized," as parents often said, "I thought these were the ups and downs of adolescence." The suicide completers frequently disclosed their suicidal thoughts to someone, usually a friend, who promised secrecy. Additionally, these teen suicide victims engaged in far more preparatory behavior than teens who attempted but did not complete suicide. Furthermore, suicide victims frequently had problems with impulsive aggression—that is, the tendency to react impulsively with hostility or aggression in response to provocation or frustration. About one-third had also made homicidal plans or threats in the week prior to death. The most common method of suicide was with a gun. Most of the increase in the teen suicide rate was in suicides by firearms, and guns were present more often in the homes of suicide completers than in those of matched controls. Their family members had very high rates of depression, substance abuse, and suicidal behavior.

One would think these interviews would be depressing; certainly the pain of the families was palpable. However, I was learning that it *was* possible to do something about adolescent suicide. We *could* improve the empirical risk assessment; we could also do a better job of recognizing depression and educating people that mood problems with impaired functioning are *not* just the normal ups and downs of adolescence. The fact that many of these teens told people about their suicidal thoughts prior to their completed suicide highlights the importance of early detection and intervention. Their friends, understandably, did not know how to respond. However, we could educate teens *not* to keep such a confidence about a friend's suicidality. Additionally, the predominant attitude among professionals was to dismiss teen suicidal talk as merely "attention seeking." Professionals often labeled medically "nonlethal" suicide attempts as "gestures," despite the teens' high suicidal intent. In fact, such ideation and behavior may well be the first step in a journey resulting in a fatal outcome. Furthermore, due to the high rates of familial suicidal behavior, collaborating with our adult colleagues could help us identify the high-risk offspring of the parents they were treating. Finally, the high rate of suicide by firearms indicated the importance of asking families to remove guns from their homes when there was a youth with high suicidal risk living there.

The net result of this work was that we now had a framework for evaluating suicidal risk. It also led to three other lines of inquiry: understanding the impact of suicide on the social network of the teen, understanding how suicide might run in families, and developing treatments for youth at risk for suicide in order to attenuate the risk.

It is hard to convey the degree of hysteria about suicide contagion that existed in those days. I recall that Kim Puig-Antich thought it was an area unworthy of study … that is, until we had our very own suicide epidemic here in Pittsburgh. Within 18 days, there were three suicides and seven suicide attempts in a local high school. We thought the people most likely to imitate suicidal behavior were those most closely exposed to the suicidal person—the teen's social network (close friends and family). We conducted a research study in which we interviewed the parents, siblings, and friends of suicide victims, as well as friends of friends. To our surprise, friends and siblings were *not* at increased risk for imitation. In fact, after adjusting for the fact that friends and siblings had much higher rates of psychiatric problems than the general population, close contacts of adolescent suicide victims were about *half* as likely as matched controls (unexposed teens) to attempt suicide. Friends of the suicide victims said that although they may have considered suicide in the past, they would never again do so, following their experience of its painful aftermath. These results helped to shape our recommendation to the media regarding how to report on the topic of completed suicide: to discourage imitation, media reports should highlight suicide as an outcome of psychiatric illness that is treatable rather than romanticize the act or the victim, which tends to heighten the likelihood of imitation.

However, the suicide did have long-lasting effects on the teen's social network. Almost one-third of the friends and siblings developed clinical depression after the suicide. The most vulnerable were those who knew of the victim's plan, had talked to the victim within 24 hours of the suicide, and felt responsible for the death. This underscores the importance of educating teens not to keep a friend's confidence about suicide. In short, the friends and family of the suicide victims were devastated for a long period after the suicide—exhibiting high levels of grief even 6 years later.

In 1986, around the time our research group was conducting the psychological autopsy studies, Kim Puig-Antich, the chief of child psychiatry and my direct supervisor, decided that we needed a teen suicide prevention program. Initially, I was reluctant to set up such a clinic. My conversation with Kim went something like this:

> KIM: David, you need to set up a clinic for suicidal teens.
>
> DAVID: But I don't know anything about treating suicidal teens.
>
> KIM: That's fine, then you'll learn!
>
> DAVID: But no one knows anything about treating suicidal teens.
>
> KIM: Great! Then no one can criticize you! Now go out and save some lives!

Although there was little known about the assessment and treatment of suicidal teens to guide us, Kim encouraged us to move forward because of the increasing problem of teen suicide. Subsequently, he brokered a partnership between me and Dr. Mary Margaret Kerr, a faculty member in the University of Pittsburgh Departments of Psychiatry and Education. We put together a proposal to the Commonwealth of Pennsylvania for a teen suicide prevention center, and the Commonwealth has generously supported that program to this very day. The program has two main components: (1) outreach, which is primarily educational and preventive, and (2) clinical, focused on intervention for suicidal youth. Within outreach, Mary Margaret developed programs for educating teachers and school administrators about how to recognize and respond to suicidal risk, as well as how to deal with the aftermath of a teen suicide in a school. My role was to conduct the research and run a clinic for suicidal teens. As soon as we learned something new from our research, Mary Margaret would translate it into training and education for thousands of education and mental health professionals.

In the clinic, we were evaluating nearly one new suicidal adolescent every day. There were no empirically validated treatments for this population, so we relied on knowledge gained from our psychological autopsies: these teens were depressed, hopeless, impulsive, and poor problem solvers. At that time, tricyclic antidepressants were the only class of medications available, had not been demonstrated to be effective for children, and were fatal in overdose. So, we elected to treat these teens with psychotherapy. We turned to the adult literature for guidance and found that Beck's cognitive therapy model effectively addressed suicidality in depressed adults. Therefore, I undertook to learn and adapt this model. Applying Beck's framework, we helped teens recognize that when depressed, they look at the world in a way that reinforces their negative mood—that is, ignoring positives, magnifying negatives, and (especially for suicidal teens) engaging in black-and-white thinking, with the ultimate dichotomy being the choice between life and death.

It was at this time, while moonlighting at a local mental health center, that I met Kimberly Poling—a bright, energetic young social worker with a natural ability to connect with adolescents. I was particularly impressed with Kim's ability to engage reluctant teens in treatment. In cases where others would have thrown up their hands in frustration, Kim's optimism and proactive approach to rapport building and collaborative problem solving yielded impressive results. Kim also demonstrated a strong desire to learn. One day when I was talking with Kim about my work at WPIC, she shared with me the information that she spent most of her Sunday afternoons at WPIC's library! She too seemed to be looking for the music that had yet to be written. I invited Kim to join me as a therapist at the teen suicide prevention program, which by then was known as Services for Teens At Risk, or STAR.

Kim joined my staff of three other therapists, and together we developed empirically informed assessment procedures, as well as treatment guidelines based on Beck's cognitive-behavioral model. We felt the treatment worked quite well, but there was one big problem: a dropout rate of around 40%. We called families who had dropped out of treatment to find out what they liked and did not like about the treatment. We found that the parents were angry with their teens and felt manipulated by their teens' suicidal behaviors. We realized we had failed to convey that their children had a disease that was not entirely in their control. Subsequently, Kim and I developed a workbook designed specifically for parents that explained the current understanding about mood disorders and teens. The workbook, *Teen Depression: A Survival Manual for Families,* provides psychoeducation on symptoms, causes, and treatments of depression and, most importantly, on how depression affects the entire family. Specific tips are offered on how the family can help the depressed teen. We started a psychoeducational/support parent program based on the workbook. Not only was the program effective in teaching parents about adolescent depression, it also led many parents to recognize and seek treatment for their own depression. This intervention was associated with a dramatic decrease in the dropout rate.

We decided to test this new cognitive-behavioral therapy (CBT) against two other credible and widely used treatments—family therapy and supportive therapy. We found that CBT was superior to the other two treatments for reducing depressive symptoms. These findings led to the recognition of CBT as an effective treatment for adolescent depression. We also found that depression improved more with CBT than with supportive treatment for teens with suicidality (current or past). However, in terms of reduction of suicidal thoughts and behavior, CBT was no better than the other two treatments. This illustrates an important theme—the apparent disconnect between the treatment response for depression and that for suicidal behavior. We also saw this clinically—a child's depression would be improving with treatment, and suddenly he or she would show up in the emergency room after an impulsive suicide attempt. When we asked what happened, he or she would describe becoming overwhelmed by intense emotions, what we have come to refer to as *emotion dysregulation.* This seemed to be an important treatment target that we had been overlooking. This led us to invite Marsha Linehan to WPIC in 1996 to conduct an intensive dialectical behavior therapy (DBT) training. The emotion regulation and distress tolerance skills we learned from Dr. Linehan complemented our treatment approach. As we implemented the integration of CBT, DBT, and family involvement at the STAR Clinic, we quickly realized this combined treatment was what we had been looking for.

Over the next several years, clinicians at the STAR Clinic implemented the treatment model, with good results. As the treatment community became aware of our success in treating depressed, suicidal teens, we began to get several requests for trainings and workshops. We heard others echo our prior concerns, that often CBT alone was not enough. We realized we had something unique and special that other clinicians could benefit from—so began our desire to write this book.

This was where Tina Goldstein entered the picture. As a doctoral student at the University of Colorado, her work with pediatric bipolar patients had led her to identify this same construct, emotion dysregulation, as an important area for assessment and treatment in pediatric mood disorders. She joined us at WPIC for her predoctoral internship, during which time she completed a 6-month clinical rotation with our teen suicide prevention program. It was immediately obvious to us that we had found a like-minded clinician and researcher. In addition to having a natural rapport with teens, she also demonstrated the rare skill Kim has aptly labeled the "bob and weave" of collaborative empiricism—that is, the ability to blend the art of clinical work with the data from empirical study while being in the moment with a patient. Tina signed on as a postdoctoral fellow under my research mentorship and Kim's clinical supervision in 2003.

Meanwhile, we were trying to understand more about contributors to risk for suicidal behavior above and beyond depression, since treating depression alone did not always eliminate risk. One way to understand risk factors for a condition is to examine their aggregation in families. In 1985, I assessed a boy who had made a serious suicide attempt. When I took a family history, it turned out his family was loaded for suicide; months later his younger brother was referred following a serious attempt. It made me wonder if there was also a genetic predisposition to suicide, above and beyond the genetic risk associated with psychiatric disorders such as depression.

To address this question, we examined the aggregation of suicide, suicidal behavior, and psychiatric disorder in the families of adolescent suicide completers and controls. The relatives of the suicide completers had a much higher rate of suicidal behavior, even after controlling for the differences in psychiatric disorder. In other words, something besides psychiatric disorder was being transmitted in these families. Our study identified the construct *impulsive aggression* as a key trait involved in the transmission of suicide risk in families. The higher rate of suicidal behavior in relatives of completers was found in families of the more aggressive suicide victims.

It is difficult to disentangle the sequence of risk retrospectively. If suicidal behavior truly runs in families, then we should be able to see this increased risk in the children of adult suicide attempters. In collaborative work with Dr. John Mann and colleagues at the New York State Psychiatric Institute, we compared the risk of suicide attempts in the offspring of adults with depression and a history of a suicide attempt to the offspring of those with mood disorder and no attempt. Despite the fact that the two offspring groups had the same rates of mood disorder and every other condition, the children of the attempters had a sixfold higher rate of attempt. One of the main factors that differentiated the two groups of children was higher levels of aggression. Furthermore, those adult attempters with the most family loading for suicidal behavior were the most aggressive, and had children who were more highly aggressive, and had children with higher rates of attempts, as well as attempts at earlier ages. This strongly suggests that the trait of impulsive aggression is important in explaining the familial pattern of suicidal behavior. It also suggests the need to develop interventions that target this trait, since it seems to be highly related to suicide risk.

This leads us to the challenges we face today. We now have treatments for teen depression that work, but they are efficacious only around 60% of the time. Consequently, we conducted a study to test alternative treatments after the initial treatment with a selective serotonin reuptake inhibitor had failed to resolve the depression, and found that the combination of CBT and medication was most effective in achieving response to depression. We have also identified genetic and pharmacokinetic factors that predict a favorable response, which may enable us to match patients with the right treatments for them.

A second challenge is that we have not yet identified treatments in adolescents that reliably prevent reattempts in individuals who have already attempted suicide. The treatment package we have developed over the years at STAR served as one of the foundations for the psychotherapy approach utilized in the multisite Treatment of Adolescent Suicide Attempters (TASA) study, which helped to establish the feasibility of delivering this treatment to geographically and ethnically diverse populations. However, like all other treatments for teens attempting suicide, it has not been definitively established as being effective. Working on the TASA project with other leading psychotherapy researchers (such as Greg Brown, John Curry, Betsy Kennard, Barbara Stanley, and Karen Wells) helped us to more carefully examine and articulate what we thought were the active ingredients in the treatment of depressed, suicidal adolescents.

At the outset of this journey, the adolescent suicide rate was going up, we had no knowledge of risk factors for suicide, there was great concern about suicide contagion, and we had no treatments for adolescent depression. Currently, the adolescent suicide rate has declined, we have an empirical framework for assessing suicidal risk, and we have several empirically validated treatments for adolescent depression. At present, there are multiple ongoing studies to identify genetic risk factors for suicidal behavior, develop interventions to target risk for recurrent suicidal behavior and resistant depression, and to prevent the onset of suicidal behavior before it starts. Yet even before the answers to these questions unfold, we can and must apply what we know in the best way we can, in order to help depressed young people who want to take their own lives. In this book, we wish to show how to best use our current knowledge to help our patients appreciate the preciousness of life and make the most of this great gift.

Our intent is to weave clinical wisdom and collaborative empiricism together into one integrated whole. We begin by reviewing assessment of depression and suicidality, and what is known about evidence-based treatments for these conditions. We then describe what we view as the necessary ingredients for the successful treatment of depressed suicidal adolescents and discuss the development of the therapeutic relationship, safety planning, and creation of a case conceptualization for treatment. Next we outline our approach to treatment, including forming a collaborative therapeutic relationship, specific treatment techniques, and helping those adolescents who recover to stay well. We conclude with thoughts on future directions for the field.

CHAPTER 1

Adolescent Depression

An Overview of Assessment and Treatment

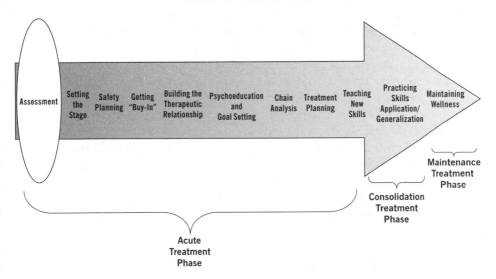

WHAT YOU WILL LEARN IN THIS CHAPTER

- Classification of different types of mood disorders.
- Assessment and differential diagnosis.
- An overview (efficacy, indications, modes of action, and adverse effects) of current treatment approaches for depressed adolescents, including psychotherapy and antidepressant medication.
- What comprises an adequate trial of an antidepressant (dose and duration).
- Suicide risks of use compared to the benefits of antidepressants.

In this chapter, we first review the diagnostic criteria for adolescent mood disorders, describe an approach to assessment and differential diagnosis, and present an overview of evidence-based treatments for depression. Then we provide the therapist with an approach to the treatment of adolescent depression.

WHY IS ADOLESCENT DEPRESSION AN IMPORTANT PROBLEM?

Depression is the psychiatric disorder that is most closely related to suicidal ideation and behavior. Around 80% of adolescent suicide attempters and 60% of adolescent suicide completers have a mood disorder. Furthermore, even when suicidal ideation or behavior is not a big part of the clinical picture, pediatric depression is a serious and common problem. Around one in five adolescents will experience at least one depressive episode before adulthood. While the disorder is twice as common in females, it is a significant source of disability for males as well. Untreated, depressed adolescents are more likely to abuse substances, have difficulties establishing and maintaining close personal relationships, and underachieve in academic and occupational domains. Adolescent depression is the gateway to recurrent or chronic depression in adults, so the proper management of depression during adolescence may make a big difference in the adolescent's long-term development.

COMMON QUESTIONS FAMILIES ASK ABOUT DEPRESSION (AND SOME BRIEF ANSWERS)

- *How common is this condition?* In any given year, about 8% of female adolescents and 3% of male adolescents will experience a serious episode of depression.
- *What causes depression?* Depression is an illness, and it runs in families. There are changes in brain circuitry and brain chemistry associated with depression that affect the depressed person's ability to regulate his or her mood and to experience positive emotions.
- *How long does this last?* Untreated, a depressive episode usually lasts around 4–8 months. However, a depressed person who is not treated will often continue to have some residual symptoms afterwards.
- *Will it come back?* Often, the depression will come back. Recurrence can often be prevented by continued treatment.

- *Will my child be able to function normally again?* With complete relief of symptoms, depressed youth do return to their previous level of functioning.
- *Why are assessment and classification important?* The assessment of depression is the key to the development of a treatment plan. There are specific recommended treatments for different types of mood disorders (examples include depression, bipolar disorder, and seasonal affective disorder). Differentiating among these mood disorder diagnoses requires careful assessment. Depressive disorders also share features with other classes of psychiatric conditions that require different treatment approaches, including anxiety disorders and attention-deficit/hyperactivity disorder (ADHD). Depression also co-occurs with other disorders that affect the patient's functioning, suicidal risk, and response to treatment for depression (e.g., substance use disorders). Finally, ongoing assessment is needed to monitor whether treatment is having an effect.

CLASSIFICATION

Mood disorders are characterized by alterations in mood that cause functional impairment; these can consist of either excessive sadness or euphoria. There are three main dimensions of mood disorder classification: polarity, severity, and chronicity.

Polarity refers to the direction of the mood change. Patients with *unipolar* depression experience "down" moods only. These dips in mood are characterized by sadness, anhedonia (i.e., the inability to have fun, often described by teens as boredom), and/or irritability. Patients with *bipolar* spectrum disorders (including bipolar I, bipolar II, bipolar not otherwise specified [NOS], and cyclothymia) experience mood swings that are extreme in both directions—down and up. The "up" moods are referred to as mania (the more severe form, seen in bipolar I) and hypomania (a less impairing form of mania, seen in bipolar II). Mania is characterized by an elevated, expansive, or irritable mood. Irritability is so common in so many adolescent psychiatric disorders that the *Diagnostic and Statistical Manual of Mental Disorders*, fourth edition, text revision (DSM-IV-TR; American Psychiatric Association, 2000) requires additional symptoms to ensure that the symptom of irritability is associated with mania, as opposed to another psychiatric disorder for which irritability is a diagnostic criterion.

Severity of the mood disorder refers to the degree of impairment it causes, its pervasiveness, and the number of associated symptoms. *Chro-*

nicity refers to the duration of the individual's symptoms. To illustrate, mania is more severe than hypomania, and DSM-IV-TR criteria require that a person's symptoms last longer in order to meet criteria for mania as opposed to hypomania. Major depression requires more symptoms for a greater proportion of the day than is required for dysthymic disorder. Forms of depression and bipolar disorder that do not meet either the symptom count or duration criteria are designated by the term *not otherwise specified* (NOS), meaning that the individual has most but not all of the features of the condition, and that the symptoms do cause functional impairment.

Two additional features of mood disorders—a seasonal pattern and psychosis—have important treatment implications. Some individuals experience depressions that have their onset or become worse in the fall. Such seasonal depressions can be treated with exposure to a certain frequency of light. Patients with psychosis also require different treatment. We discuss how to assess for these conditions below.

Depressive Subtypes

Major depression is the most severe of the unipolar depressive disorders (for full criteria, see American Psychiatric Association, 2000). A diagnosis of dysthymic disorder requires fewer symptoms than major depression. Furthermore, the symptoms do not need to be as pervasive in dysthymia (i.e., a majority of the time, as compared to nearly all of the time in major depression). Despite its lesser symptom criteria, therapists should not be fooled by this condition—it is quite impairing due to its chronicity. Patients with dysthymic disorder often cannot recall ever feeling happy. Often, dysthymia develops into a full-blown major depressive disorder. The occurrence of major depressive disorder with dysthymic disorder is termed double depression, and is common in individuals presenting with depressions that are treatment resistant.

CASE EXAMPLE

A therapist conducted a feedback session for parents following the assessment of their 14-year-old daughter, Ann. Ann's mother reported that her daughter seemed to have good days interspersed with days when she would be down, hopeless, and withdrawn. Based on this inconsistency, Ann's mother expressed her belief that Ann was just trying to get attention. Ann's report was consistent with her mother's observation. At the same time, Ann said she could not recall a time when she felt good for as long a 3 days in a row. How might the therapist respond to Ann's mother's observation?

RESPONSE

Ann has dysthymic disorder, a diagnosis consistent with both Ann's and her mother's observations. The therapist might explain that Ann has a chronic but intermittent depressive disorder that will not likely remit on its own without treatment.

Bipolar Disorder in Adolescents

The current DSM adult criteria are probably not adequate to diagnose bipolar disorder in adolescents, because the illness tends to present differently in children and adolescents than it does in adults. Youth with bipolar disorder present with fewer clear, distinct episodes of mania and depression. Instead, adolescents with bipolar disorder may experience rapid cycling, in which manic and depressed moods alternate rapidly (several times within a week, or even within a day). Consequently, youth with bipolar disorder often do not fulfill the DSM duration criteria. Also, youth with bipolar NOS or bipolar II disorder have a high probability of eventually developing bipolar I, whereas that is not the case among adults.

A major depressive episode in an individual with bipolar disorder can be indistinguishable from a major depressive episode in someone with unipolar disorder. Research studies show that patients with psychotic depression are more likely to develop bipolar disorder, as are those with a family history of bipolar disorder. Every depressed adolescent patient should be screened for a history of mania or hypomania, and monitored prospectively for the development of manic symptoms. Clinicians should also carefully assess for a family history of bipolar disorder, since a parental history of bipolar disorder increases the risk to the child more than tenfold. Distinguishing unipolar from bipolar depression in adolescents is challenging. In both conditions the individual can present with mood lability and irritability. However, in the case of unipolar depression, the lability does not include cycling into hypomania. Irritability alone is not specific to bipolar disorder; rather, to meet criteria for hypomania, diagnostic symptoms must present in clusters and include other cardinal hypomanic and manic symptoms (e.g., grandiosity, hypersexuality, and excessive joking).

Now that we have established the definitions of the different mood-related conditions, we can discuss how to assess them.

GUIDELINES FOR ASSESSMENT
OF MOOD DISORDERS

- *Look for the core symptoms.* First, the therapist should inquire about mood changes, both down and up. Without sadness, anhedonia, or irritability, a person will not meet criteria for a depressive disorder. Without an expansive or elevated mood, a person will not meet criteria for a bipolar spectrum disorder.

- *Have the patient use his or own words to describe mood.* In assessing for depressive symptoms, it is critical to make sure that the therapist and the teen have a common vocabulary. One way to accomplish this is to have the teen describe, in his or her own words, the experience of negative mood—for example, "blah," "numb," irritable," "bored," "no fun," or "sad." Often, adolescents will already have a vocabulary for describing their symptoms. The therapist can then use those terms when talking with the patient about his or her symptoms, and when tracking mood.

- *Assess for specific mood symptoms.* It is helpful to get some idea of how severe the teen thinks his or her mood symptoms are—for example, the clinician can ask, "On a scale of 1 to 10, if 10 is the best you have ever felt, how would you rate your mood now? How would you describe a '10'?" In assessing anhedonia, one can ask, "What do you do for fun?" If the teen says, "Now, nothing," then the therapist can find out what he or she used to do for fun, and then ask what is different now—for example, one can ask, "Could you tell me about the last time that you had a really good time? How would you compare that to [a time before you were depressed]?" Patients who have been in treatment may appear to be symptom-free due to the absence of depression. However, they may lack the ability to experience happiness, well-being, or joy. These youth are at risk for a recurrence because the experiences of mastery and pleasure are protective against the development of depression.

- Mania can be assessed by asking, "Have you ever had an experience of being really 'up,' feeling on top of the world, with a whole lot of energy?" Euphoria, grandiosity, hypersexuality, and excessive joking are other specific indicators of mania. Irritability is a possible criteria for mania, but without other symptoms it is very nonspecific. If the patient answers in the affirmative, then the therapist should ask about the most recent time this happened and have the patient describe the experience in detail. Even depressed youth can have some good days, and the therapist will want to distinguish between being "depression-free" and manic. As is the case in discussing depression, the therapist and patient should try to find common terminology to describe manic symptoms, for example, "high," "up," "feeling on top of the world," or "super." Often adolescent patients with bipolar spectrum disorders experience rapid mood cycling. The adolescent should be asked to consider how his or her moods change within one day. Also, adolescents with bipolar disorder often experience mixed states, meaning that they meet criteria for both mania and depression at the same time. This is a very dangerous situation because they have the impulsivity and energy of mania combined with the dysphoria and pessimism of depression, putting them at very high suicidal risk.

• *Use a time line to establish onset, time course, and fluctuations in mood.* We encourage the therapist to start by drawing a time line with the patient as a means of "visualizing" the course of his or her mood problems. The time line for fluctuations in mood can be an incredibly helpful tool for establishing the course of mood symptoms and their association with comorbid disorders. In creating the time line, it is helpful to use temporal markers that will be meaningful to the patient, like holidays, vacations, social events (e.g., homecoming), or the beginning or end of school. The time line can also help the therapist to determine if a given symptom is attributable to depression, or whether it is more likely related to some other condition (e.g., a learning disorder).

The therapist can begin by having the teen draw out the rough course of his or her mood fluctuations since the symptom onset (see Figure 1.1). Fluctuations can then be tied to other mood-related symptoms, life events, comorbid conditions, and changes in treatment.

CASE EXAMPLE

A 16-year-old boy, Aaron, was brought in by his parents postdischarge from the hospital after making a very medically serious suicide attempt. He said that he now feels "fine" and does not need treatment. Aaron did disclose that he quit football a couple of weeks before his attempt, even though he was one of the stars of the team. How could the therapist use this information to clarify Aaron's diagnostic status?

RESPONSE

The therapist asked what Aaron's experience of football was last year, and if he noticed anything different about how things have gone this year. Aaron replied that this year he felt like he was just going through the motions at practice. He stated that he thought the coach was starting him just because he felt sorry for him, and Aaron felt he had actually become a drag on the team—all very different from his experience the year before. When the therapist

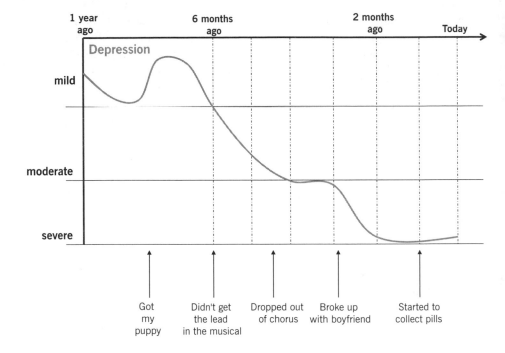

FIGURE 1.1. Sample time line of depression symptoms.

asked Aaron how he felt during his football practices, he became angry and said, "Numb! Numb! Everyone keeps thinking that I am depressed, but really I can't feel anything at all!" Now the therapist has discovered how to talk about Aaron's depressive episode with him, using his own language.

These principles are summarized in Figure 1.2.

Assessing Sleep

Sleep problems are commonly seen in adolescents with mood disorders and include difficulty falling asleep or staying asleep, and early morning awakening; conversely, some adolescents report sleeping too much, napping during the day, and always feeling tired. Suggested questions for assessing sleep difficulties are presented in Figure 1.3. If the patient has difficulty falling asleep, the therapist should find inquire about the patient's bedtime routine. Is the patient lying in bed ruminating about the day, or is he or she using technology late at night (e.g., computer,

- Inquire about the core symptoms.
- Ask the patient to describe each symptom in his or her own words.
- Assess for specific symptoms.
- Determine the time course, intensity, frequency, and contribution to impairment for each symptom.
- Assess if the symptom could be accounted for by other circumstances or another disorder.
- Before making a diagnosis, verify that symptoms of the disorder cluster together in time.

FIGURE 1.2. Basic guidelines for assessment of mood disorders.

phone)? There may be other factors contributing to difficulty with sleep onset and/or quality; for example, use of caffeinated beverages, afternoon napping, and a change in medication type or dose can impact sleep. Use of a stimulant or bupropion (Wellbutrin) can cause difficulty sleeping. Similarly, selective serotonin reuptake inhibitors (SSRIs) can cause sleep disruption and vivid dreams that can disturb sleep. The antipsychotics, although usually sedative, can sometimes cause restlessness that interferes with sleep.

A person with bipolar disorder may have difficulty falling asleep. However, when manic, the individual does not need or even want to sleep, and will not feel tired the next day. In fact, sleep deprivation, if anything, can precipitate or increase manic symptoms in patients with a bipolar disorder. In contrast, those with unipolar depression will report feeling tired and irritable following nights with little or no sleep.

- "What is your bedtime routine?"
- "What time do you go to bed?"
- "How long does it take you to fall asleep?"
- "Do you sleep through the night?"
- "When do you wake up?"
- "Do you sleep during the day?"
- "Do you drink anything with caffeine?"

FIGURE 1.3. Assessing sleep.

CASE EXAMPLE

Rayna, 16, presented for an evaluation for declining grades and depressed mood. She reported taking more than 2 hours to fall asleep. When asked about her sleep routine, Rayna stated that she routinely stays up until 1 in the morning completing her homework, and then has trouble "turning off [my] brain." Moreover, she was taking naps each afternoon and drinking a cup of coffee in the evening prior to starting her homework. Should the evaluator consider Rayna's sleep difficulty a symptom of depression?

RESPONSE

Not at this point. Upon further questioning, it became apparent that the reason for Rayna's routine was that she was taking all Advanced Placement courses and was having trouble keeping up with all of the work. Further assessment should focus on whether the workload is just too hard for anyone, or whether there was a decline in Rayna's functioning. In the meantime, Rayna was advised to stop taking naps and drinking coffee late at night.

Assessing Appetite and Weight

Depression can be associated with either increases or decreases in appetite and weight. Such changes in weight need to be evaluated taking into account normal growth, since maintaining the same weight during a period of growth for an adolescent is equivalent to weight loss in an adult. Weight loss and appetite loss associated with depression should be distinguished from intentional weight loss for someone who is dieting, or restrictive eating for a patient with an eating disorder. Another consideration is whether a medical condition or medication may be affecting weight and appetite. Patients frequently lose weight taking bupropion, and often initially when taking SSRIs. Long-term use of antipsychotics, and to a lesser extent SSRIs, is associated with weight gain (see Figure 1.4).

Assessing Concentration and Decision Making

When asking the teen about his or her capacity to concentrate, one might ask, "Have you noticed that you have been having more difficulty doing your homework, or focusing in school?" It is important to rule out other reasons for difficulty with schoolwork such as taking an overly ambitious courseload, being bullied, or having ADHD or learning disabilities. If the concentration problems began with the onset of ADHD,

---

- "Have you noticed a change in your appetite, either up or down?"
- "Has there been any change in your weight?"
  - If yes: "Are you trying to gain/lose weight?"
  - If yes: "What is your target?"
  - If target is unrealistically thin, pursue questions about eating disorder.

FIGURE 1.4. Assessing appetite and weight.

then they need to have worsened in the face of mood problems in order to be included in the symptom count for depression. A bright student who is depressed may be able to continue to perform well but may have to work much harder to keep up. If such a student has kept his or her grades up, the therapist might also ask, "Do you have to work harder now to achieve the same success?" One aspect of depression that may interfere with concentration is rumination—that is, continued preoccupation, often about a perceived slight, that interferes with optimal concentration on a given task.

Assessing difficulty making decisions is fairly straightforward, for example, "Do you notice that you have difficulty making decisions?" If the teen responds that he or she does, then the therapist can follow up with "Could you give me examples of some decisions you have had to make lately? How has that gone?"

CASE EXAMPLE

Jason is a 16-year-old with a history of ADHD. He was referred for an evaluation for depression after turning in an essay in English class that was very self-deprecatory. In it, Jason indicated that he was sad about his lack of achievement, especially as he was seeing his friends prepare for college. In the evaluation, Jason confirmed difficulty concentrating in school, although he reported that he has had problems concentrating in school ever since kindergarten. How might the therapist determine whether Jason's difficulty concentrating is associated with depression?

RESPONSE

The therapist should first determine whether Jason has other symptoms of depression. Then, the therapist should ascertain whether there was any change in Jason's ability to concentrate or make decisions associated with changes in mood. The therapist could ask

Jason specifically what he noticed about his ability to concentrate around the time that he turned in the essay. After further questioning, Jason felt there was no change in his ability to concentrate, so the difficulty concentrating is most likely related to his long-standing ADHD.

Assessing Feelings of Worthlessness and Guilt

Depressed patients often feel that they are a burden to others, and that they have little in the way of redeeming features. However, other psychiatric conditions can also lead to feeling unworthy—for example, a patient with a learning disability who does not experience school success, a patient who is overweight and whose parents berate her about her weight, or a patient with an eating disorder who won't feel good about herself until she hits a certain target weight. Patients with obsessive–compulsive disorder (OCD) may also experience pathological guilt; however, guilt in OCD is usually about inappropriate thoughts, or about failing to complete a complex ritual that involves purification or cleanliness. Sometimes psychotic depression manifests itself with delusions about sinfulness, worthlessness or somatic delusions. Some suggested questions for assessing self-worth and guilt are presented in Figure 1.5.

Assessing Psychosis

One cannot just look at a patient and tell whether or not he or she is having psychotic symptoms. Therefore, it is important to specifically ask about these symptoms. If the patient appears guarded or paranoid, it is best to begin by asking if he or she is concerned about something, or was bothered by any of the questions. The therapist can explain, "I am

---

- "Can you tell me three good things about you?"
- "What about three not-so-good things?"
- "Do you think you are important to others?"
- "Do you consider yourself a burden on others?"
- "Have you done things for which you feel guilty?"
- "When you do something wrong, what goes through your mind?"
- "What kinds of things make you feel guilty?"

FIGURE 1.5. Assessing self-worth and guilt.

going to ask some questions that might seem odd, but they are important because they might help us to understand what is going on with you." Such items include (1) thoughts that people are out to get him or her; (2) ideas that others are trying to read or control his or her mind; (3) hearing voices or seeing things; or (4) specific negative ideas, like being possessed by the devil, having an incurable disease, having committed a great sin, or thinking the world is coming to an end. If a patient answers yes to any of these items, a follow-up question could be "Are you convinced this is true, or do you doubt it?" The therapist should also inquire about the patient's reaction to these thoughts. When a patient says that he or she is hearing voices, the therapist can ask if the voice seems different than his or her own thoughts, whether the voice is real or in the patient's imagination, whether it is consistently a specific person, and whether the thoughts are speaking to him or her or making certain requests or demands. In general, the more certain the person is that the phenomena are real and that he or she has to respond to them, the more likely the experience is one of psychosis. Psychosis can be part of the presentation of depression, mania (in which case it is usually dominated by grandiosity and paranoia), or schizophrenia. In the latter case, some common first signs of schizophrenia resemble symptoms of depression (e.g., changes in mood, social withdrawal, and difficulty concentrating). See Figure 1.6 for suggestions regarding assessment of psychosis.

- "Have you had the experience of your mind playing tricks on you? Have you heard voices talk to you or about you? Do you have ideas others might consider unusual?"
- "Have you felt that people are talking about you or following you?"
- "Do you ever think that you can control other people's thoughts, or that they can control yours? How about the radio or TV?"
- "Do you ever have ideas about having special powers, or being chosen for a special task, a unique reward, or a special punishment?"
- "To what extent do you feel that these [see above] are real, and to what extent due to your own thoughts or imagination?"
- "To what extent can you tune these thoughts out?"
- "To what extent do you feel the need to act on these thoughts [e.g., if command hallucinations]?"

FIGURE 1.6. Assessing psychotic symptoms.

CASE EXAMPLE

A 14-year-old girl presented after a suicide attempt with depressed affect and was extremely guarded. She said that she was hearing voices telling her to kill herself. She tells the assessing clinician that she will not answer too many more questions. What should the clinician ask?

RESPONSE

It seems likely that the patient is psychotic. Differential diagnosis is neither possible nor is it the first priority under these circumstances. Rather, the clinician should aim to assess the aspects of her psychotic symptoms that are most likely to put her in danger. Two possible questions are "Are the voices still telling you to kill yourself?" and "How likely are you to follow their instructions?" Another might be "what can you do to keep yourself safe?"

DIFFERENTIAL DIAGNOSIS AND ASSESSMENT OF COMORBIDITY

Table 1.1 lists the key symptoms of depression, and how other common diagnoses can be distinguished from depression. In addition, it is important to be aware that these conditions are commonly comorbid with depression, and their role in the patient's functioning and recovery from depression may be important. In the case of comorbidity, the diagnostic time line can be used to highlight the interrelationship among different disorders. In this section, we review how to distinguish other common disorders from depression, how to disentangle the role of each condition in outcome, and how these comorbidities affect treatment planning.

Anxiety Disorders

Anxiety disorders can affect mood, sleep, and concentration. However, as compared to depressive symptoms, anxiety symptoms are often relieved if the patient can avoid the anxiety-provoking situation. A patient with social phobia is concerned about his or her worthiness in the eyes of others, whereas a patient with depression has a low view of his or her own self-worth.

Anxiety disorders frequently precede and are comorbid with depression. The use of the time line to chart changes in anxious and depressive symptoms can help to determine if one is dealing primarily with a

TABLE 1.1. Differential Diagnosis of Depressive Symptoms

Symptom	Anxiety disorder	ADHD	Substance use	OCD	Eating disorder
Mood	Low mood when forced to face anxiogenic situation	Irritability, mood instability due to stimulants, demoralization due to school/peer issues	Can cause euphoria or depression, but temporarily related to use	Low mood if unable to complete ritual, or disturbed about unacceptable thoughts	Low mood due to nutritional issues or because being made to maintain a certain weight
Concentration	Difficulty concentrating due to rumination	Difficulty since early childhood	Memory, motivation, focus can be affected during and after use	Can be impaired due to intrusive thoughts or need to do rituals	Usually OK, but can be affected by nutritional status and preoccupation with weight
Sleep	Difficulty falling asleep due to worrying	May be disturbed due to stimulant	Can cause sleep disruption or hypersomnia	If have comorbid tics, or if rituals or thoughts interfere with sleep	Secondary to nutritional status; may either have excessive exercise or fatigue
Appetite	Usually not affected	May be affected by stimulant, but should be OK after medication wears off	Can cause increase or decrease	If thoughts/rituals related to food	Down, but associated with body image distortion and restrictive eating patterns. In bulimia, binging and purging
Worthlessness/guilt	Worried that others will think he or she is not worthwhile	May have poor self-esteem from continued failure in school and with peers	May experience remorse postintoxication, especially after getting in trouble	Feel ashamed of thoughts, guilty about not completing rituals	Low self-worth associated with dissatisfaction with weight or with binging/purging

depressive disorder, an anxiety disorder, or both. Comorbid anxiety can affect the outcome of treatment for depression, since the anxiety may interfere with the pursuit of pleasurable activities and mastery that are necessary for a full recovery.

Obsessive–Compulsive Disorder

The symptoms of OCD, which is classified as an anxiety disorder in DSM-IV-TR but has some unique characteristics, often overlap with depression. Those who have socially inappropriate obsessive thoughts may feel ashamed and guilty, and have difficulty concentrating. Patients with paralyzing rituals may be limited in their ability to engage in enjoyable activities, and may feel guilty, anxious, and sad if they are unable to accomplish the rituals successfully. Depression often co-occurs with OCD. By using a diagnostic time line, the clinician can discern whether the symptoms of depression are secondary to manifestations of OCD or represent an independent disorder.

Posttraumatic Stress Disorder

Posttraumatic stress disorder (PTSD) is also currently grouped with the anxiety disorders in DSM-IV-TR but also has distinctive characteristics. It can affect concentration and mood, cause irritability, interfere with the ability to enjoy oneself, and result in sleep disruption. PTSD and depression are frequently comorbid because similar stressors (e.g., abuse, assault, bereavement) increase risk for both. The mood symptoms of PTSD are more likely to be triggered or exacerbated by a traumatic reminder.

Bereavement

Normal bereavement understandably results in sadness and withdrawal. Current diagnostic guidelines make it very difficult to diagnose depression in bereaved individuals, which we think is a mistake. Stress can precipitate depression in a vulnerable individual, and there are very few events more stressful for an adolescent than the loss of a parent. If a patient presents with functional impairment and symptoms of depression, particularly if there has been a past personal or family history of depression, then the diagnosis of depression is reasonable. Depression can also be confused with complicated grief, which involves intense preoccupation with the loss, anger and bitterness, pining for the deceased, numbness, intrusive images and memories, and avoidance of things that

remind the person of the deceased. along with functional impairment
on and complicated grief occur
remit unless the issues related to

ood, concentration, sleep, appe-
th ADHD can become demoral-
rejection; occasionally, stimulant
ptoms. Concentration is an obvi-
e onset of ADHD is usually much
We would only expect symptoms
develops depression. Youth with
n, and be able to compensate for
ir school career, when academic
1 occur due to the accumulated
es. In addition, ADHD is often
c time line is useful for mapping
ed with each disorder over time.
may indeed experience depres-
lifficulties. If the impulsivity and
onally impairing symptoms, then
ADHD first, and then reevaluate

ic every symptom of a mood dis-
xication, the immediate afteref-
fects, or the longer-term consequences. If the patient is not forthcom-
ing about his or her use, then urine or blood testing for substances is
often the only way to identify this diagnostic category. Other clues to the
role of alcohol and substance abuse are a change in school attendance
patterns, switching to a new set of friends known to be involved with
alcohol and drugs, and behavioral changes that seem to follow social
gatherings.

Alcohol and drug use frequently co-occur with depression, and each
increases risk for the other. In addition to the pharmacological effects
of alcohol and drugs on depressive symptoms, substance use increases
the chances of events with disciplinary or legal consequences that can
precipitate a depression. Use of alcohol and drugs while in treatment for

depression makes response to treatment less likely. Patients sometimes are more likely to report alcohol and substance abuse on self-report questionnaires than when asked directly by the clinician. Also, any patient who has not responded to evidence-based treatment, barring another explanation, should be tested for alcohol and drugs.

Eating Disorders

Individuals with restrictive eating disorders who are nutritionally compromised may have many symptoms of depression. The patient may be sad and have low self-worth because she does not meet her impossible standards of thinness, or because she is being forced to gain weight. Patients with bulimia may experience sadness, poor self-worth, and guilt, but it is often related to shame about body image and purging. However, depression and eating disorders frequently co-occur. The clinician should give priority to the condition that is most relevant to the patient's survival and functioning. For individuals with bulimia and comorbid mood disorders, it is helpful to use a diagnostic time line to determine if the bulimia is a mode of coping with the depression (in which case the depression is primary), or if the depression occurs as a consequence of the bulimia. In cases where the two conditions are temporally intertwined, primacy may be determined by the degree of distress caused by symptoms and the patient's own priorities.

In addition to assessing for depression and comorbid conditions, the therapist should also assess for other treatment targets (e.g., other patient and family characteristics; see Table 1.2) that, if unaddressed, may contribute to a poorer treatment response.

TABLE 1.2. Important Domains to Assess with Depression in Adolescents

Domain	Impact on treatment for depression
Abuse/bullying	Poorer response to combined psychotherapy and medication treatment
Family conflict	Poorer and less complete response to any form of treatment; higher risk for relapse
Comorbidity (anxiety/ADHD)	Better response to combined treatment
Alcohol/substance use	Poorer response to combined treatment
Maternal depression	Poorer response to CBT

AN OVERVIEW OF EVIDENCE-BASED TREATMENT OPTIONS FOR ADOLESCENT DEPRESSION

This section provides the information a therapist needs (1) to help a patient and family give informed consent to treatment, and (2) to match patients with specific treatments. The treatment approaches described below, which have been proven effective in the treatment of adolescent depression, are cognitive-behavioral therapy (CBT), interpersonal therapy (IPT), antidepressant medication, and the combination of CBT and medication. Because this book takes a CBT perspective, we will not discuss IPT further, except to say that while it has not been as widely studied as CBT, it seems to be an excellent treatment. In our discussions of both CBT and antidepressant medication, we describe the treatment and how it works, summarize how well it works compared to other treatments, discuss how to match the treatment to the individual patient, and discuss the risks of the treatment.

Cognitive-Behavioral Therapy

What Is CBT?

CBT is a treatment that focuses on the relationship between depression and how individuals think about the world, themselves, and the future. CBT is a time-limited treatment in which the therapist is active and directive. The relationship between the therapist and patient in CBT is best defined as what Dr. Aaron T. Beck termed *collaborative empiricism*. CBT includes a wide range of therapeutic techniques that are based on two simple principles: (1) There is a close interrelationship among thoughts, emotions, and behaviors, and (2) distressing emotions associated with a disorder such as depression can be relieved by altering patterns of thinking and behavior.

The goal of CBT is to help the patient identify, explore, and modify the patterns of negative thinking that lead to depression and problematic behavior. However, in practice, sometimes the focus of intervention in CBT is not the patient's thoughts, but his or her behaviors. This treatment focus on changing behavior in order to trigger changes in thoughts and emotions is referred to as *behavioral activation*. An alternative treatment focus includes emotions. For patients who become very emotionally distressed, the therapist and patient may choose to work on improving emotion regulation and distress tolerance skills. Treatments that emphasize this approach include a specialized type of CBT called dialectical behavior therapy (DBT). In our treatment of depressed and

- Mood monitoring
- Behavioral activation, pleasant activity scheduling
- Cognitive restructuring
- Relaxation and stress management
- Emotion regulation and distress tolerance
- Social skills and conflict resolution
- General problem-solving skills

FIGURE 1.7. Common elements of cognitive-behavioral therapy (CBT).

suicidal adolescents, we incorporate elements of DBT into our CBT approach. In subsequent chapters, we explain in more detail how to implement the different components of CBT for depressed and suicidal youth; common techniques are outlined in Figure 1.7.

CBT approaches vary in the degree of structure that is recommended. Some are highly structured and didactic, with the therapist following a standard order in teaching skills and techniques to patients. While results from studies using this type of CBT approach are good, our approach is more closely modeled on the work of the founder of CBT, Dr. Aaron Beck. This CBT treatment approach is more flexible, and the modules and techniques are chosen collaboratively with the patient and family and tailored to the patient's needs. The advantage of the more structured CBT approach is that all patients receive a standard, quality-controlled treatment. The advantage of our more flexible approach is that we are empowering the patient to take responsibility for his or her care. We tell our patients, "We are going to teach you to become your own therapist." This less structured approach is accepted well by teens, who often have some ambivalence about being in treatment in the first place.

What Is a Reasonable Dose of CBT?

Most studies have used at least 12 sessions of CBT, but there is some suggestion that to get to remission and to prevent relapse, you need to use more sessions than just 12.

What Are the Stages of CBT?

There are three stages in this model of CBT: acute, consolidation, and maintenance treatment (see Figure 1.8). In this approach, movement

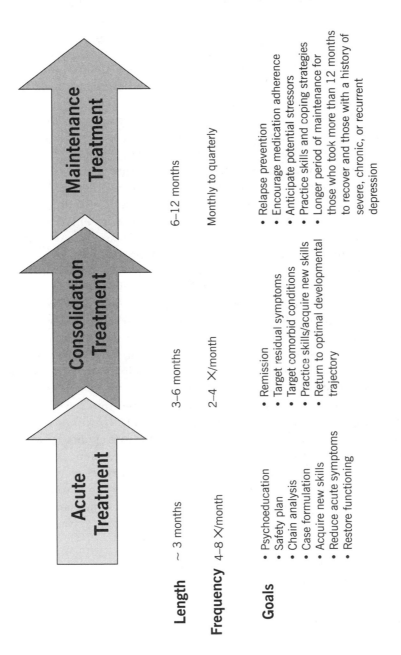

Acute Treatment → **Consolidation Treatment** → **Maintenance Treatment**

Length ~ 3 months | 3–6 months | 6–12 months

Frequency 4–8 X/month | 2–4 X/month | Monthly to quarterly

Goals

Acute Treatment:
- Psychoeducation
- Safety plan
- Chain analysis
- Case formulation
- Acquire new skills
- Reduce acute symptoms
- Restore functioning

Consolidation Treatment:
- Remission
- Target residual symptoms
- Target comorbid conditions
- Practice skills/acquire new skills
- Return to optimal developmental trajectory

Maintenance Treatment:
- Relapse prevention
- Encourage medication adherence
- Anticipate potential stressors
- Practice skills and coping strategies
- Longer period of maintenance for those who took more than 12 months to recover and those with a history of severe, chronic, or recurrent depression

FIGURE 1.8. The three stages of treatment of adolescent depression.

from one stage of treatment to the next is prompted by achievement of the treatment goals of the preceding stage. We provide rough guidelines for stage length and frequency of sessions in Figure 1.8.

This book primarily emphasizes strategies to be employed during the acute phase of treatment. The primary goals of acute treatment are to establish the patient's safety, create and pursue an individualized treatment plan, and stabilize acute psychiatric symptoms. During acute treatment, the therapist and patient work toward achieving a clinical response and the restoration of functioning. The second stage of treatment, consolidation, involves solidification of the therapeutic gains that have been achieved. The goal of the patient and therapist in this stage is to move from response to remission—that is, the complete absence of depressive symptoms. The main outcome in most clinical studies is *clinical response,* meaning that the patient is *better.* It does *not* mean that the patient is *well.* The achievement of remission after response takes time, and often, additional treatment. The consolidation stage of treatment also includes targeting of residual difficulties that are likely to result in a recurrence if unaddressed. The third and final stage of treatment is maintenance. The goal of maintenance treatment is to prevent the return of depression. The risk of relapse or recurrence is highest within the first 4 months after the patient has gotten better, and patients who continue with medication and/or psychotherapy are the most likely to stay well. Another focus of maintenance is to help the patient anticipate upcoming stressors that could lead to a recurrence. Additionally, patients identify and strengthen skills and strategies they have learned that will help them cope with upcoming stressors. During maintenance treatment, patients are encouraged to focus on lifestyle changes that will help sustain their recovery. Finally, maintenance treatment is encouraged for those patients with a history of severe, chronic, or recurrent depression, as well as for those patients whose recovery took more than 12 months. During this extended follow-up, prevention of relapse is targeted.

What Evidence Supports the Use of CBT for the Acute Treatment of Adolescent Depression?

Part of treatment is education about the benefits and risks of each treatment. We briefly summarize the "bottom line" results from studies examining how CBT compares to other forms of treatment, as follows:

1. CBT helps patients get better faster than other types of acute therapy (supportive, relaxation, family therapy) and is roughly equivalent to the effects of IPT, the other evidence-based psychotherapy for adolescent depression. About 6 in 10 depressed youth will show a favorable response to CBT.
2. Medication alone gets patients better faster than CBT alone, although by 18 weeks, CBT has caught up to medication.
3. Medication plus CBT provides the best results, and obtains them the fastest. Medication plus CBT is better than medication alone, and much better than CBT alone during the first 12 weeks of treatment.
4. Depressed youth continue to improve beyond 3 months of treatment, so persistence is important.
5. There are a lot of people who do not respond even to the "best" treatment. We believe that by individualizing treatment, addressing concomitant problems that are often not targeted in research studies, and being persistent it is possible to improve upon these results.

For Whom Is CBT Particularly Advantageous?

CBT is particularly effective in comparison to other treatments in patients who are more complex diagnostically—such as those with comorbid anxiety, ADHD, or conduct disorder. For patients with many cognitive distortions, CBT would seem to be a good fit, but if a patient with severe depression appears particularly "stuck" in his or her distortions, then CBT will work best in combination with antidepressant medication. CBT requires that the patient monitor his or her mood and practice skills learned in the session during the week. A patient who is unwilling or unable to do so is less likely to benefit.

For Whom Is CBT Not as Effective?

Patients with a history of physical or sexual abuse do not tend to do well with CBT, either alone or in combination with medication. Patients whose motivation or concentration is impaired due to severe depression may do better with medication alone until they achieve some symptom relief. There are also environmental factors that may interfere with any credible treatment, namely current maternal depression, family discord, or bullying at school. CBT is less likely to be effective until these issues are addressed.

Individualizing Treatment

For patients with chronic and/or severe depression, combination treatment is superior to medication alone in terms of speed of response, which is an important consideration in a depressed, suicidal patient. Furthermore, known environmental stressors such as maternal depression or family conflict need to be addressed early in treatment. In addition, the choice of which CBT skills to use with a particular patient and family is dependent on the nature of the presenting problems and goals.

Antidepressant Medication

Medication and the Role of the Nonmedical Therapist

Most therapists who work with depressed and suicidal adolescents do not have prescribing privileges. Nevertheless, patients, families, and nonpsychiatric physicians look to the therapist for advice about whether to start medication or adjust the dosage, and to assess side effects. Furthermore, if the patient is being treated with medication, then the nonmedical therapist must be able to incorporate that information into his or her assessment, and be informed enough about antidepressants and their use to be able to effectively collaborate with prescribing clinicians. Therefore, we provide information about antidepressants that is likely to be useful to a nonmedical therapist whose patient is receiving medication. Some basic dos and don'ts for patients are listed in Figure 1.9.

What Are Antidepressants?

Antidepressants are drugs used to treat depression. These drugs are frequently used to treat anxiety disorders as well. Table 1.3 lists some

Do:	Don't:
• Take your medication every day. • Report any side effects. • Tell other healthcare providers that you are on this medicine. • Check with a pharmacist and MD before adding any other medications. • Avoid alcohol and drugs.	• Stop medication abruptly. • Change dosage without talking with your clinical team. • Think that medication is the answer to all your problems. • Have surgery without telling the surgeon you are taking an SSRI.

FIGURE 1.9. Dos and don'ts for patients taking antidepressants.

TABLE 1.3. Antidepressants Used to Treat Adolescent Depression

Generic name	Trade name	Class	Dose	Half-life
Fluoxetine*	Prozac	SSRI	20–60 mg	5 days
Escitalopram*	Lexapro	SSRI	10–40 mg	16–24 hours
Citalopram	Celexa	SSRI	20–60 mg	12–24 hours
Sertraline	Zoloft	SSRI	50–150 mg	15–20 hours
Venlafaxine	Effexor XR	SNRI	150–300 mg	11 hours
Bupropion	Wellbutrin XL	Increase synaptic norepinephrine and dopamine	300–450 mg	16.5 hours
Duloxetine	Cymbalta	SNRI	20–60 mg	12 hours

*These are the only two medications that are FDA-approved for use in adolescent depression.

of the antidepressants most commonly used for adolescent depression, the range of commonly used dosages, and the half-lives of these medications. The half-life is the time it takes for half the medication to be cleared from a patient's system; adolescents tend to metabolize drugs more quickly than adults.

How Do They Work?

The brain consists of circuits of nerve cells. Two nerve cells (or neurons) communicate is across a synapse by releasing and taking up chemicals that either activate or damp down the activity in a neuron. The most commonly used antidepressants in pediatric depression are the selective serotonin reuptake inhibitors (SSRIs). These drugs increase the availability of serotonin in the synapse. Two SSRIs are approved by the U.S. Food and Drug Administration (FDA) for use in adolescents: fluoxetine (Prozac) and escitalopram (Lexapro). Escitalopram is the active ingredient in citalopram (Celexa), another commonly used antidepressant. Sertraline (Zoloft) is often used for the treatment of depression, although its effects have the strongest evidence for OCD and other anxiety disorders. A second type of antidepressant acts on two important neurotransmitter systems—serotonin and norepinephrine—and is referred to as a serotonin–norepinephrine reuptake inhibitor (SNRI). Two drugs in this class are venlafaxine (Effexor) and

duloxetine (Cymbalta). Other antidepressants primarily increase norepinephrine availability; these include bupropion (Wellbutrin).

What Evidence Supports the Use of Antidepressants in the Treatment of Adolescent Depression?

Overall, depressed youth who get antidepressants are more likely to
show a clinical response compared to youth treated with placebo. About
6 in 10 depressed adolescents will show a good clinical response to an
SSRI.

Are Some Drugs Better Than Others?

The medication that has the strongest performance is fluoxetine, which
showed a much bigger difference between drug and placebo than most
of the other medications tested. However, the main difference between
these studies is that the nonfluoxetine studies have very high placebo
response rates. The fluoxetine studies were the most carefully done and
probably screened out people likely to respond to placebo. Paroxetine
does not seem to be efficacious and we no longer use it for the treatment
of adolescent depression.

Since fluoxetine and escitalopram are both FDA approved, we initiate treatment using either one of these medications. If a patient has a
personal or family history of intolerance of a medication, we will then
start with a different SSRI, like sertraline.

Which People Will Antidepressants Be Most and Least Likely to Help?

The effect of antidepressants on depression seems to be stronger for
adolescents than for children, except for studies using fluoxetine, in
which the results are similar. In general, the more severe the depression,
the bigger the difference between medication and placebo. In the large
multisite Treatment of Adolescent Depression Study (TADS) (March et
al., 2004), the more severe the depression, the more significant was the
effect of medication compared to placebo and CBT.

Patients with a definite or suspected bipolar depression should be
carefully evaluated and considered for treatment with a mood stabilizer
like lithium, divalproex, or an atypical antipsychotic prior to the initiation of antidepressant treatment. Those with a family history of bipolar
disorder should be treated first with psychotherapy, given the increased
risk for developing mania with antidepressant treatment.

What Is an Adequate Trial of an SSRI or Other Medication?

It takes about 4 weeks to be able to tell if a patient is going to respond to a given dosage of an antidepressant. We usually start at one-half the usual dose for 1 week, followed by 3 weeks of exposure at an "entry level" dosage. At that point, if there has not been a satisfactory response and there are no side effects, we would recommend increasing the dosage. If the patient has been adherent and been exposed to an entry-level dosage and one increase and has shown no improvement, this would be considered an adequate trial and a switch in medication is recommended.

Are Some Medications Better for Some Patients Than Others?

We wish we knew the answer to this question. In the meantime, we try to go by whatever clues we can gather, such as whether another family member did well, or could not tolerate a particular antidepressant. It is not really known why a patient will do well with one SSRI and not another. In any case, about half the people who do poorly on one SSRI will do well on another one.

Can an SSRI Cause Someone to Commit Suicide?

Looking across all the studies of pediatric depression, the risk of a suicidal event (i.e., increased suicidal ideation, getting ready to make an attempt, or actually making a suicide attempt) was about 3% in those who were given drug and 2% in those given placebo, a slightly but significantly increased risk. In over 4,300 youth exposed to antidepressants in clinical trials for depression and anxiety, there has not been a single suicide. Those most at risk for a suicidal event come into the study with suicidal ideation.

Is the Benefit of Using an SSRI Worth the Risk?

The number of youth who will respond to an antidepressant is 11 times higher than the number of youth who will experience a suicidal event. Also, there is a risk of suicide from untreated depression while CBT is also effective, in the TADS, CBT did not catch up to medication for 18 weeks. That is a really long time in the life of an adolescent—practically half of a school year. Thus, getting that patient better more quickly could have really important long-term implications. Plus, the longer the patient remains depressed, the longer he or she is at risk for suicidal behavior.

What Can Be Done to Minimize the Risk of Suicidal Events When Using Antidepressants?

Suicidal events tend to occur early in treatment, with the median time to an event around 3–6 weeks. We recommend seeing patients weekly for the first 6 weeks after the initiation of treatment with an antidepressant. We also recommend increasing the dosage gradually. We develop a safety plan (see Chapter 4), and review it at each visit. We tell patients and families about the risks, and ask that they contact us right away if they notice anything different and concerning about the patient's mood, thoughts, or behavior. Since one of the risk factors for suicidal events is continued depression, we often recommend a combination of CBT and medication, which results in the most rapid response.

CASE EXAMPLE

A depressed adolescent patient has just been started on an antidepressant. How often should he be seen?

RESPONSE

The risk for a suicide event is highest in the first 3–6 weeks after the initiation of antidepressant treatment. During that time, the patient should be seen weekly. If weekly visits are a hardship due to distance, then the patient should be monitored over the phone. The patient should be taught to self-monitor for sudden shifts in mood, increased irritability or lability, agitation, difficulty sitting still, and of course, changes in the frequency, intensity, or severity of suicidal ideation. Any change within a week of initiation or a medication dose change should be considered related to medication until proven otherwise. In addition, the therapist should have developed a safety plan with the patient and family to be implemented if the patient experiences an increase in suicidality.

What Are Some of the Other Side Effects Associated with the Use of SSRIs?

We list the most common side effects in Figure 1.10. Many of the physical side effects such as abdominal discomfort and headache are transient, so if possible, the patient should be encouraged to wait these out unless they prove too debilitating. Patients should be cautioned about stopping the drug abruptly because withdrawal symptoms, including flu-like symptoms, anxiety, and agitation, may occur.

Physical symptoms	Psychiatric symptoms
• Headache	• Agitation/restlessness
• Abdominal discomfort	• Anxiety
• Loss of appetite	• Fatigue
• Increased appetite	• Sleep disruption
• Easy bruising	• Vivid dreams
• Sweating	**More rarely:**
	• Irritability
	• Worsening depression
	• New onset of or worsening suicidal ideation
	• Mania

FIGURE 1.10. Side effects of SSRIs.

Medication, Psychotherapy, or Both?

The main advantage of medication over psychotherapy is that it requires less time and effort, and results in a more rapid response. The disadvantages are the potential side effects of medication, the most serious of which is a slightly elevated risk for increased suicidal ideation or behavior. The main advantage of psychotherapy is that it is not associated with any of the side effects of medication, and in theory, the skills learned in psychotherapy can be used to prevent further episodes. The main reason to use both medication and psychotherapy at the same time is that the acute response and remission rates are the highest for individuals who receive both. For chronic, recurrent, or severe depression, it makes sense to implement both treatments at the same time, since the goal is to get the adolescent functioning as soon as possible.

What this means is that while the bulk of the evidence supports use of combination treatment, especially for more severe or chronic depression, one can find support for using medication alone and, in other studies that did not involve medication, for using CBT alone. In formulating a treatment plan with the patient and family, there are data that support starting with CBT, medication, or the combination. Therefore, if the patient and family have a strong preference, it makes sense to initiate that particular treatment modality and reassess the patient in 4–6 weeks.

KEY POINTS

- Assessment of depression and comorbid conditions can be facilitated by the use of a time line.

- CBT and SSRI antidepressants are both efficacious treatments for adolescent depression.

- Although SSRIs do seems to increase the risk for suicidal ideation and behavior, the increase is less than 1%, and 11 times more depressed youth benefit from medication than experience a suicidal event.

- The combination of CBT and an SSRI is most effective, especially for those with chronic and severe depression.

- Regular follow-up and assessment of progress and side effects are key elements of treatment.

- The treatment of an episode of depression typically has three stages: acute, consolidation, and maintenance treatment.

CHAPTER 2

Assessment and Treatment of Suicidal Ideation and Behavior

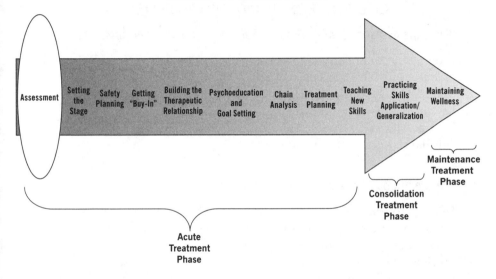

WHAT YOU WILL LEARN IN THIS CHAPTER

- Definitions of suicidal and self-injurious behavior.
- Important domains to cover in assessment of a suicidal adolescent, in order to formulate a treatment plan.
- How to determine imminent suicidal risk and the proper level of care.
- General principles in assessment of suicidal youth.

43

In this chapter, we provide definitions of different types of suicidal thoughts and behavior, describe the likelihood that one type of suicidal behavior will progress to a more severe form, suggest some general principles for the assessment of suicidal risk, and identify five key domains of inquiry. For each domain, we define it, explain why it is important, and describe how it should be assessed. Finally, we provide a framework for the assessment of imminent suicidal risk and determination of the appropriate level of care.

SIGNIFICANCE OF SUICIDAL BEHAVIOR AND SOME IMPORTANT DEFINITIONS

Why Is the Assessment of Adolescent Suicidal Behavior Important?

Over 5,000 American adolescents die by suicide each year, making suicide the third leading cause of death among adolescents in the United States. Almost all adolescents who complete suicide have shown some psychiatric disorder, and many have had previous suicidal ideation or have previously attempted suicide. Therefore, the proper assessment of suicidal risk can be life-saving.

The Spectrum of Suicidal Ideation and Behavior

In order to communicate effectively with other treatment providers and family members, it is important to use accepted terminology for the classification of suicidal thoughts and behavior (Posner et al., 2007). Suicidal ideation and behavior can be thought of as a spectrum from passive thoughts of death to the more serious form of suicidal behavior, completed suicide (see Figure 2.1). It is important to identify where along the continuum a patient currently falls, because the current level of suicidality is a strong determinant of an assessment of suicidal risk. Suicidal behavior should be distinguished from nonsuicidal self-injury (NSSI). NSSI involves stereotyped and repetitive self-harm (such as superficial cutting), with the goal not to die, but to relieve negative emotion or obtain social reinforcement. Often suicidal adolescents also engage in NSSI.

Sucidality at the lowest end of severity is the most common and least likely to progress to more serious manifestations of suicidal behavior (Figure 2.2). The less specific and intense the suicidality, the more common it is, and the less likely it is to progress to a more serious manifestation of suicidal behavior. About one in five adolescents have fleeting sui-

- *Passive death wish:* Thoughts of own death without any intent to act on it.
- *Suicidal thoughts without plan or intent:* Thoughts of attempting suicide without a concrete plan or intent to actually engage in suicidal behavior.
- *Suicidal thoughts with plan and/or intent:* Thoughts of suicide with a plan to commit suicide and/or intent to carry this plan out.
- *Suicidal threat:* Verbal expression to another person of suicidal intent.
- *Interrupted attempt:* Takes preparatory steps to engage in suicidal behavior, but stops self.
- *Aborted attempt:* Takes preparatory steps to engage in suicidal behavior, but another person unexpectedly intervenes and stops the attempt.
- *Suicide attempt:* Self-destructive behavior with explicit or inferred intent to die.
- *Suicide completion:* Suicide attempt that results in fatality.

FIGURE 2.1. The continuum of suicidal ideation and behavior.

cidal thoughts without intent or plan, but only 6% at any one time have a suicidal ideation with a plan. About half of those with a plan will go on to make a suicide attempt within a year, but many others make a suicide attempt without a long period of consideration. About 3% of male and 8% of female adolescents make a suicide attempt each year, and of these, around one in four will make a reattempt, most commonly within 6 months of the first attempt. While the majority of suicide attempters will not go on to complete suicide, the risk of suicide is still 30–60 times higher among attempters than in the population at large.

Suicidal thoughts without plan or intent	20%
Suicidal thoughts with plan and/or intent	6%
Likelihood that those with ideation with a plan will make an attempt within 1 year	50%
Proportion of adolescents who make a suicide attempt in 1 year	3–8%
Risk of reattempt within 1 year	15–30%
Risk of completed suicide among suicide attempts within 1 year	0.5–1.0%

FIGURE 2.2. The frequency and course of adolescent suicidal ideation and behavior.

CASE EXAMPLE

A 14-year-old girl who attempted suicide was discharged from a psychiatric hospital, and given an outpatient appointment in 3 weeks. Is this a reasonable follow-up plan? Why or why not?

RESPONSE

The peak time for reattempt is shortly after the initial attempt. In this case, the highest risk for reattempt is *before* the time of follow-up outpatient appointment. Therefore, the outpatient appointment should be much sooner in order to be consistent with what we know about the natural history of suicidal behavior.

GENERAL PRINCIPLES FOR ASSESSMENT

Assessment Is the Beginning of Treatment

Assessment is the beginning of the therapeutic process. Ideally, the person conducting the thorough assessment will also be the treating therapist. As in any therapeutic interaction, the clinician should explain the rationale behind the assessment questions. If the patient looks reluctant, the therapist should explore concerns rather than pushing ahead. In the beginning of the assessment, the patient should be given an overview of the topics to be covered in the assessment. The main purpose of assessment is to guide treatment. Each aspect of the assessment is used to determine level of care, degree of suicidal risk, and areas to be targeted in treatment.

Use Open-Ended Questions

In the assessment process, no matter how collaborative the mindset of the clinician, the relationship between the assessor and the patient is very unequal, and consequently, it is easy to put words in the patient's mouth. Asking open-ended questions rather than those that can be answered "yes" or "no" will provide much more information. Often, the clinician will even obtain answers to questions he or she did not even plan to ask. For example, it is preferable to ask, "How hopeless did you feel at that point?" as compared to "Were you hopeless?" In trying to assess the events, feelings, thoughts, and symptoms related to a suicidal event, it is usually helpful to have the patient tell his or her story as a first step. Then the clinician can go back and try to clarify details that fill in the different domains that we believe are most important (we describe these domains in detail below).

Ask Permission

The therapist should not only explain to the patient why a particular topic is important, but also ask if it is OK to inquire about it. This is particularly true for emotionally charged issues like sexual orientation, previous trauma, or the events leading up to a suicide attempt.

Monitor Nonverbal Behavior

Skilled clinicians continuously monitor nonverbal behavior. If a patient suddenly becomes nervous or shows an abrupt shift in affect, it is useful to check out if a particular question made the patient feel uncomfortable, or if there is more that he or she wants to add. In these instances, it can be helpful to note aloud the observed behavior—for example, "It appeared that I just said something that may have made you feel uncomfortable. I am wondering what just happened for you?" Sometimes the discrepancy between the patient's report and his or her nonverbal behavior can be telling; for example, the patient may say that a particular event had no meaning to him or her, but blushes when discussing it. Also, one can look for overall consistency between different types of information. If a patient denies having symptoms during a period of time when his or her grades are plummeting and he or she has withdrawn from activities that were formerly important, then the clinician should probe further—for example, "Can you help me understand what factors contributed to your dropping grades and your decision to quit band and gymnastics during this past semester?"

FIVE KEY DOMAINS OF INQUIRY

We recommend five key domains that the clinician should assess in order to develop a comprehensive treatment plan (see also Figure 2.3):

1. Characteristics of current and past suicidal ideation and behavior.
2. Psychiatric disorder.
3. Psychological traits.

4. Family/environmental stressors and supports.
5. Availability of lethal methods.

Each of these areas contributes to suicidal risk, meaning that a particular factor (e.g., suicidal ideation with a plan) is more common in those who go on to attempt or complete suicide. We describe each domain, explain why it is important to assess, provide sample assessment questions, and discuss the responses in terms of treatment planning and assessment of suicidal risk.

Domain 1: Characteristics of Current and Past Suicidal Ideation and Behavior

We identify seven areas relevant to suicidal ideation and behavior that should be assessed: (1) severity, frequency, and intensity of suicidal ideation; (2) reasons for living; (3) suicidal intent; (4) lethality; (5) motivation; (6) precipitant; and (7) environmental response to the suicidal behavior.

Severity, Frequency, and Intensity of Suicidal Ideation

WHAT?

Severity refers to the degree to which the person experiences suicidal ideation that is focused on specific suicidal behavior—that is, thoughts about intent and a specific plan. *Frequency* of suicidal thoughts refers to what proportion of the day a patient thinks about suicide. *Intensity* refers to the extent to which an individual is preoccupied with suicidal thoughts, and cannot distract him- or herself from them.

---

1. Current and past suicidal ideation/behavior.
2. Psychiatric disorder.
3. Psychological traits.
4. Family/environmental stressors and supports.
5. Availability of lethal methods.

FIGURE 2.3. Five key domains to assess in suicidal adolescents.

WHY?

A common misconception in assessing suicidal individuals is that people who talk about suicide do not actually take action. In fact, adolescents who complete suicide are much more likely than adolescent suicide attempters or community controls to have expressed suicidal thoughts to someone. Expressing suicidal plans out loud is an indication of the intensity of suicidal ideation.

Patients with suicidal ideation who have a specific plan and an intent to carry out the plan are the most likely to actually make an attempt within the next year. Patients with higher frequency and intensity of suicidal ideation are most likely to act on their suicidal urges. High frequency and intensity of ideation often go hand in hand with a high degree of planning and intent. Most people have had fleeting passive thoughts about death at some time; however, these do not have much clinical importance. In general, suicidal ideation is most concerning if it is frequent, of high intensity, and associated with planning and intent.

This is not to say that suicide or suicidal behavior cannot occur without previous evidence of ideation. In fact, many adolescents attempt suicide without much forethought. This is most commonly found in adolescents who are impulsive and/or are intoxicated during the suicidal act.

Sometimes an adolescent will express suicidal thoughts to a friend and ask for confidentiality. In our studies of the aftermath of adolescent suicide, the friends of the suicide victims who had known about the victims' plans and told no one were likely to have long-term difficulties with grief, depression, and PTSD. Futhermore, keeping the confidence did not help the victims. We learn two additional lessons from this. First, teens should be taught to go to a responsible adult if a friend confides that he or she is contemplating suicide, because "it is better to lose a friendship than a friend." Second, the fact that these suicide victims were confiding in other people prior to their deaths meant that their suicides were potentially preventable, because at least in part, they wanted to be discovered and saved. Even in these highest-risk individuals, the wish to live and the wish to die can coexist.

HOW?

The clinician should first probe for the type of suicidal ideation that the patient is experiencing (nonspecific, ideation with a plan, intent, etc.;

- "Have you ever thought you would be better off dead?"
- "Have ever had thoughts of taking your own life?"
- "Have you ever made a plan to commit suicide?"
- "Have you ever had the intent to carry out your suicidal urges/plans?"
- "Have you ever attempted suicide?"
- If answer to any question is positive, ask for examples, and establish if current, recent, or ever. Also elicit information about the most serious episode ever.

FIGURE 2.4. Assessing suicidal ideation and behavior.

see Figure 2.4). Once the type of ideation the patient is experiencing is identified, the clinician should probe the issues raised in Figure 2.5 to clarify the frequency and intensity of ideation. The clinician can assess frequency by asking, "What proportion of the day do you find yourself having suicidal thoughts?" or "In a given hour, how much of the time are you having thoughts of suicide?" *Intensity* refers to the extent to which the suicidal thoughts represent a preoccupation that intrudes upon, or dominates, an individual's consciousness. Another way to refer to intensity is "suicidal urges." One may inquire by asking, "On a scale of 1 to 10, if 10 represents total preoccupation and 1 represents no thoughts whatsoever, where would you place yourself?" Finally, there is the aspect of intent and planning. Adolescents who have suicidal ideation with a concrete plan are much more likely to carry it out within a year. Intent and planning can be ascertained by asking, "When you have suicidal thoughts, to what extent do you plan to act on them?" or "Do you have a specific plan?"

- "For what proportion of the day do you find yourself having suicidal thoughts?"
- "In a given hour, how much of the time are you thinking about suicide?"
- "To what extent can you push away the suicidal thoughts and think about something else (on a scale of 1–10 scale, if 1 is easy to push away, 10 is completely preoccupied)?"
- "To what extent do you feel you can resist suicidal urges (on a scale of 1–10, if 1 is completely, 10 is not at all)?"

FIGURE 2.5. Assessing frequency and severity of suicidal ideation.

CASE EXAMPLE

A 13-year-old boy, Greg, was being disciplined by his teacher. Greg told his teacher that if he was punished, he was going to kill himself. The school ordered that Greg receive a psychiatric evaluation. Greg's parents thought that their son was just trying to get out of his punishment. How can the clinician determine whether this was just "something he said," or whether Greg is really at increased risk for suicide?

RESPONSE

The clinician can ask Greg what he meant when he said he was going to "kill himself." Did he have a plan and intent? Did he have suicidal thoughts in the past? If so, how frequently? If Greg answers that he has never had such thoughts before, has no plan or intent, is functioning well at home and in school, and that it was just "something he said," then it is important to educate both Greg and his parents about the seriousness with which such statements should be taken. We recommend seeing Greg and his family for two to four additional sessions to ensure that nothing has been missed. These sessions can also be used to understand how the disciplinary situation resulted in Greg's suicidal threat.

Reasons for Living

WHAT?

Reasons for living are reasons the person with suicidal ideation reports have kept him or her from taking action on the suicidal ideation. Most commonly, patients provide reasons such as lack of "courage," not wanting to hurt parents or other loved ones, religious concerns, some hopefulness about the future, or even hopefulness about the possibility that treatment could help.

WHY?

Patients with suicidal ideation who have concrete reasons for living are less likely to attempt suicide. Hopelessness, or pessimism about the future (e.g., "Things will never work out for me," "I have nothing to look forward to," "This will never get any better"), predicts dropout from treatment, suicide attempts, and eventual suicide. Suicide attempters who have strong reasons for living are grateful for having survived their suicide attempt. Understanding what is keeping the person alive is at least as critical to the formulation of a treatment plan as knowing why the person wants to die. This highlights a very important principle in dealing with suicidal individuals: The wish to live coexists with the wish to die. Our job as mental health professionals is to help tip the balance away from death and toward life.

HOW?

The clinician should acknowledge the intensity, severity, and frequency of the patient's ideation and then ask, "What has kept you from acting on these thoughts/urges?" The clinician should also inquire about what, if anything, the patient is looking forward to in the future, and whether he or she has any hopefulness about treatment. Understanding what things keep the person from killing him- or herself and motivate him or her to live are very important. When possible, these reasons for living should be incorporated into the treatment plan (see Figure 2.6).

CASE EXAMPLE

A 13-year-old girl, Hannah, presented with depression and intense, frequent, and severe suicidal ideation. She reported that she had not acted on her suicidal thoughts because she did not want to hurt her family and because she had aspirations as a musician and an artist. Interviews with Hannah's parents confirmed that she is a talented and accomplished artist and musician, but has had little opportunity to develop these talents. What is an intervention that could help to strengthen this particular "reason for living"?

- "You've mentioned that your suicidal thoughts are pretty intense. What is keeping you from acting on these suicidal urges?"
- "You've mentioned some reasons why you are thinking of attempting suicide. What are some reasons to keep on living? Is there any way we can make that stronger?"
- "To what extent are you hopeful that treatment can help you? What would make you more/less hopeful?"
- [For those who have already attempted] "To what extent do you regret having survived? To what extent do you regret having attempted?"

FIGURE 2.6. Reasons for living.

RESPONSE

The clinician identified a free after-school arts program that Hannah could participate in, as well as a local community orchestra. As her depression lifted, Hannah was encouraged to apply to the local arts-concentration high school.

If a person has actually made an attempt, it is important to ask whether he or she regrets not dying. If a patient responds with gratitude for having survived, then it is important to understand what is sustaining his or her will to live.

The domains of intent, lethality, motivation, precipitant, and environmental response, discussed next, are most applicable to the assessment of adolescents who have made a prior suicide attempt. However, when patients have discrete episodes of suicidal thinking, the same domains apply and can be useful in the identification of appropriate treatment targets.

Suicidal Intent

WHAT?

Suicidal intent is defined as the extent to which the suicide attempter wished to die. This is assessed by directly asking the patient, but also can be inferred from the patient's behavior prior to the attempt. Factors like the degree of planning of the attempt and whether the attempt was timed in such as way as to make discovery more or less likely may give the clinician additional important information about the individual's intent.

WHY?

Adolescents who complete suicide show much greater suicidal intent than do those who attempt suicide. Additionally, suicide attempters with high suicidal intent are more likely to reattempt in the future, and also to ultimately complete suicide. In adults, suicidal intent has been shown to be related to hopelessness even more closely than to the severity of depression. In addition to assessing the degree of suicidal intent at the time of the attempt, it is also important to assess the frequency and severity of ideation after the attempt. An important question that predicts suicide reattempt and completion in adults is "Do you regret surviving your suicide attempt?" Those who express regret at surviving are at very high risk for completed suicide, especially if they do not express any countervailing reasons for living.

The suicide attempt and completion rate is much lower for children and younger adolescents than it is for older adolescents. In part, this is because younger children, due to the level of their cognitive abilities, are largely unable to plan and execute a lethal suicide attempt. Even among suicide completers, those over the age of 16 have higher suicidal intent and more evidence of planning than those under the age of 16, for whom attempts tend to be more impulsive.

HOW?

It is best to begin with open-ended questions, like "Please tell me about the events that led up to your suicide attempt." (See Figure 2.7 for further suggestions about assessing for suicidal intent.) Then the clinician can follow up with specific questions about planning and circumstances of the attempt. Sometimes adolescents deny that they wanted to die at the time of the attempt, yet their behavior indicates that they planned the attempt in such a way that death would be likely. If a patient has a mistaken idea about the high lethality of a given method (e.g., a teenager believes that taking five Advil can be fatal), then his or her choice of that method conveys high intent, even if the information is mistaken. It is best not to ask questions that can be answered with "yes" or "no." In other words, rather than asking, "Did you plan this attempt?" it is often more informative to ask "What did you do to plan for this attempt?" As described above, the clinician should ask whether the suicide attempter now regrets his or her decision, or, alternatively, is upset that he or she survived. Often, a suicidal act mobilizes family support in the short run, and the person's desire to commit suicide may temporarily subside.

- *Planning:* "What kind of planning did you do?"
- *Prior communication:* "Did you tell anyone that you were intending to commit suicide?"
- *Note:* "Did you leave a note?"
- *Likelihood of rescue:* "How did you choose the time and place of the attempt?"
- *Likelihood of fatal outcome:* "Why did you choose this particular method?"
- *Wish to die:* "To what extent did you want to die?"
- *Regret:* "Are you happy that you survived?"

FIGURE 2.7. Assessing suicidal intent.

CASE EXAMPLE

Julie, a 16-year-old girl with a history of epilepsy, became depressed after she began treatment for her seizure disorder. She stopped taking her antiseizure medication and saved up a large number of the pills over many weeks. She then took an overdose consisting of all of the pills she had saved up and ended up in the intensive care unit. When questioned about her suicide attempt, Julie claimed that it was an accident. What conclusions would one draw from this information about Julie's possible intent, and what additional questions might further clarify the situation?

RESPONSE

The number of pills Julie took, plus the long-term planning involved in stockpiling the pills, indicates that the overdose was not accidental, and that Julie showed a high degree of planning, which implies high suicidal intent. One might follow up by asking, "Are you glad that you survived?" "What might one expect to happen to someone who takes that number of these type of pills?" and "At what time of day and where did this happen?" If the patient appeared to time the attempt to avoid discovery, that would be additional information supporting the inference of high suicidal intent. This highlights the utility of the construct of suicidal intent, which relies not only on what the patient says, but also on his or her actual behavior.

Lethality

WHAT?

Lethality refers to the actual bodily damage associated with an attempt. In addition, it also refers to the *potential* medical damage associated with a method—such as a suicide attempt by gunshot that due to chance did not do a great deal of medical damage.

WHY?

Suicide attempts in which highly lethal methods are chosen (e.g., firearms, hanging, asphyxiation, or jumping) are often associated with completed suicide. Attempters who choose lethal methods but do not complete suicide are at higher risk for ultimately completing suicide, because these acts show high intent. Lethality, though, is imperfectly correlated with intent. It is for this reason that the use of the term "suicide gesture" is discouraged. There are three reasons why lethality is not perfectly correlated with intent: (1) Younger attempters (and occasionally older teens as well) may have misinformation regarding the lethality of a particular method, and thus a high-intent attempt might not result in an attempt of very high lethality; (2) a suicide attempter might use a potentially highly lethal method but somehow escape relatively unscathed (e.g., shooting that resulted in little irreversible damage); and (3) an impulsive suicide attempter might make a suicide attempt of high lethality simply because he or she either misjudged the potential lethality of the method, or because it was the most accessible. For example, a cognitively immature 12-year-old might engage in an attempt of low lethality, like trying to drown in the bathtub, but with high suicidal intent. Conversely, a 16-year-old might impulsively take a large number of acetaminophen without explicit intent to die, but the result might be liver toxicity and even death.

HOW?

The clinician should note the method, the actual medical damage, and the likelihood of death in using that particular method. The patient's perception of the lethality of the method should also be ascertained (see Figure 2.8).

CASE EXAMPLE

An 11-year-old girl, Maria, swallowed some pills from the medicine cabinet and went to her room without telling anyone. Later in the night, her mother found Maria throwing up in the bathroom. Maria then disclosed the overdose. She was taken to the local pediatric emergency room, examined, and medically cleared to go home. The clinician was called in to evaluate Maria for a suicide "gesture" to determine disposition. The medical team was eager to discharge Maria, stating that "her attempt was obviously not serious, since very little medical damage took place." What key questions should

---

- What is the likelihood of fatality with a given method?
- High-lethality methods include firearms, hanging, jumping, asphyxiation, overdose with fatal amount of medication.
- What did the patient think was going to be the result of the use of a given method?

FIGURE 2.8. Assessing lethality of suicidal behavior.

the clinician ask, and how should these be communicated to the medical team?

RESPONSE

The clinician should ask Maria what she was expecting would happen when she took these pills, to what extent she was hoping to die, and whether she is happy that she survived. The clinician discovers through this line of questioning that Maria wanted to die and regrets having been discovered by her mother. The clinician should explain to the medical treatment team that Maria's continued wish to die is concerning and that the lethality of the attempt is not a good guide to the seriousness of the attempt in young children.

Motivation

WHAT?

Motivation is defined as the end result that the suicide attempter hoped to achieve by making the attempt. Attempters frequently express more than one motivation. The most common reasons given for making a suicide attempt are to die, to escape painful affect or an intolerable situation, or to influence someone else's behavior or feelings. For example, sometimes adolescents attempt suicide to get someone to pay attention to them or to express hostility. Those patients who primarily or solely express a wish to die tend to be more depressed and hopeless than those who engage in suicidal behavior for other reasons (see Table 2.1).

TABLE 2.1. Most Common Motivations for Adolescent Suicide Attempts

Motivation	Primary reason	Any reason
Death	28%	56%
Escape mental pain	18%	57%
Escape difficult situation	13%	55%
Communicate desperation	9%	28%
To test or communicate love	7%	48%
Induce regret or fright	4%	29%
Influence someone, get help	3%	31%

Note. Data from Boergers, Spirito, and Donaldson (1998).

WHY?

Every behavior happens for a reason. Suicidal behavior is a means of meeting a need (e.g., to influence others, to express strong feelings, to escape painful emotions). If those needs are not met, then it is likely that the suicidal behavior will recur. Different motivations call for different treatment strategies, as will be discussed below. We aim to communicate to our patients that there are safer, more effective, and more efficient ways to meet our needs than by attempting suicide. Family members may express anger or label such suicidal behavior as "manipulative," particularly when the need being expressed is interpersonal. However, the word *manipulative* implies that the patient is "in control," whereas a suicide attempt indicates that the patient is out of control. Family members should be told that the treatment is designed to help the patient better identify his or her needs, and address those needs by applying skills that he or she will learn in treatment, rather than through life-threatening behaviors like a suicide attempt.

HOW?

The clinician should ask the patient, "What did you hope would be different as a result of your attempt?" or "What were you hoping to achieve by making a suicide attempt?" It is important to explain to the patient the rationale for exploring motivation: "If together we understand what you were trying to achieve, and we can find different, safer, and more effective ways for you to meet those needs, then suicidal behavior may not be such an appealing option." Frequently, patients express more than one motivation, but usually there is one that is most prominent. It is not uncommon for adolescents to have a hard time answering questions about motivation for suicidal behavior. They may not be aware of their motivations, or their motivations may lead them to feel embarrassed or ashamed. If this is the case, the clinician should take a step back with the patient and ask for a description of everything he or she can remember leading up to the suicide attempt (also see Chapter 5). Through reconstruction of the events and associated thoughts and feelings leading up to the attempt, the patient and clinician may be able to infer possible motivations—for example, "When you took the overdose, how much did you want your boyfriend to feel guilty?" It can also be helpful to ask the patient specifically but in an open-ended way about motivations that others sometimes have for suicidal behavior. Patients may find it validating to realize that others have had similar experiences.

Regardless of the motivation expressed, the therapist should validate the importance of the goal the patient tried to achieve, while also raising the possibility that there are safer and more effective ways to achieve the same ends. Patients who want to die are often hopeless, so assessment and treatment must target reasons for living and for improving hopefulness. For patients who express a wish to escape painful emotions, it is important to try to identify as precisely as possible what aspect of the patient's emotional experience is the most painful—is it anxiety, agitation, unremitting sadness? Patients who make suicide attempts are frequently global in their responses, and achieving the greatest degree of precision about what exactly is the nature of the emotional suffering will allow for more precise targeting of treatment. Treatment should focus both on improving skills (e.g., emotion regulation, toleration of distress) and on relief of psychiatric symptoms through psychotherapy and medication. If the primary motivation for a patient is to escape a painful social situation, then an exploration of that situation, its hazards, and how the patient can cope with it is warranted. Patients may describe intolerable situations like abuse at home or bullying at school, which may require removal from the home or a school intervention to stop the bullying. Sometimes the "intolerable" situation is based on the perception of the patient, such as not having a boyfriend, in which case the assessment should pursue what aspects of not having a boyfriend are intolerable. Treatment would then focus on alternative ways of viewing and coping with the intolerable situation. Another common motivation for suicidal behavior in adolescents is to express a feeling or elicit a response from someone important in their environment (i.e., to gain attention, take revenge, express hostility, or get someone to change his or her mind about something). For those adolescents who show interpersonal motivations, the clinician should explore the extent to which the patient is able to identify feelings and needs, problem-solve, express anger or disappointment directly, and effectively communicate needs and wants to another person (see Table 2.2).

TABLE 2.2. Assessment of Motivation for Attempts

Motivation	Assessment questions
To die	Hopelessness, reasons for living, regret at surviving.
Painful affect	Identify type of affect, tie to psychopathology, distress tolerance.
Painful situation	Assess for safety (abuse), bullying; identify *what* is intolerable and why.
Express feeling	Affect identification, assertiveness, communication skills.
Influence others	Ability to identify needs, assertiveness, communication skills.

CASE EXAMPLE

A 9-year-old boy, Adam, made a highly lethal suicide attempt. He was very depressed, but was not exhibiting psychotic symptoms. Adam was admitted to a psychiatric hospital. He reported that he wished he had died. He gave as his motivation a desire to "get away from here," but would not disclose anything further. What further assessment strategies could the clinician pursue in Adam's case?

RESPONSE

A highly lethal suicide attempt in a nonpsychotic child age 9 is highly likely to be related to either abuse or bullying. The clinician could look for signs of abuse or assault, and also question his parents. Upon medical examination, Adam showed evidence of anal penetration. When the clinician confronted Adam's mother with this information, she disclosed a suspicion that the stepfather in the home was abusing Adam.

Precipitant

WHAT?

The precipitant is the event or series of events that led the patient to attempt suicide. Precipitants usually occur within 24–48 hours of the attempt (exceptions include ongoing stressors like abuse). The most likely situation to precipitate suicidal behavior in younger adolescents is conflict with parents. With older adolescents, the precipitant more often involves conflict with peers. Other precipitants include school failure, disciplinary or legal problems, and disruption or loss of an interpersonal relationship. Other possible precipitants include abuse at home, a physical or sexual assault, bullying at school, or events or feelings related to recognition of same-sex attraction or orientation (see Figure 2.9).

- "Please tell me, in your own words, the events that led up to your making a suicide attempt."
- "What has happened recently that may have pushed you in the direction of wanting to make a suicide attempt?"
- "You mentioned some of the things that you were hoping to achieve [escape, get attention, etc.] by making an attempt. What caused you to decide to make an attempt now?"

FIGURE 2.9. Assessing precipitants leading up to suicide attempts.

WHY?

All suicidal patients simultaneously experience a wish to live and a wish to die. The goal of assessment is to identify those personal and environmental factors that are likely to tilt the balance away from making a suicide attempt and toward life. If the precipitants that are identified by the patient are closely related to the motivation for the initial suicide attempt and are likely to be recurrent, then an initial focus of treatment should be either on reducing the frequency and intensity of the precipitant, or modifying the patient's reaction to it. If the patient's motivation is to escape an intolerable situation, such as abuse or bullying, then the initial treatment focus for the therapy should be on eliminating this particular environmental precipitant. In other cases, the best approach may be a combination of reducing the likelihood that the precipitant will recur and changing the patient's and family's response to that precipitant. If parent–child discord about a particular issue (e.g., chores or homework) is cited as the precipitant, then the clinician may negotiate a short-term truce with regard to these "hot topics" and get permission for either party to leave the room and cool off, rather than allowing the discussion to escalate to full-blown conflict (see Chapter 4 for further information). Later in treatment, when parents and the patient have learned about more effective communication and problem-solving skills, revisiting these issues will be more productive.

HOW?

The precipitant should be explored both by asking the patient to describe the events leading up to the suicide attempt, and then by asking more specifically, "What were the most important things that happened that tipped you toward making a suicide attempt?" Sometimes patients may identify more than one precipitant. The motivation for an attempt can be a clue as to the precipitants, and vice versa. Patients who want to escape painful emotions may not identify a clear event, but instead speak to not being able to stand their continuing emotional distress. Still, one should probe further to try to understand why the person made a suicide attempt *at this specific point* if he or she had been in distress for some period of time. For patients who want to escape an "impossible" situation, some aspect of that situation (like abuse or bullying) is likely to be the precipitant. For patients with interpersonal motivations, the precipitants often involve interpersonal discord, disappointment, or loss (see Figure 2.10).

- Conflict with parents
- Conflict with peers
- Interpersonal loss or disappointment
- School difficulties
- Legal or disciplinary issues
- Abuse, assault, witnessing domestic violence
- Being bullied
- Concerns about sexual orientation

FIGURE 2.10. Common precipitants for adolescent suicidal behavior.

CASE EXAMPLE

A 16-year-old girl who made a suicide attempt says that she made her attempt because she was trying to "escape [her] problems," but is not specific, despite further probing. When asked what may have tipped her in the direction of an attempt, she is not able to identify any one event. What questions might the clinician ask to try to further understand what precipitated the suicide attempt?

RESPONSE

The clinician might back up and ask the patient to describe, in her own words, what the week leading up to her suicide attempt was like. The clinician could also ask her how long she has had these problems, and what about them caused her to make an attempt *at that particular point*.

Environmental Response to the Suicidal Behavior

WHAT?

The environmental response to the suicide attempt includes the reactions of parents, other relatives, friends, clinicians, and educators. The reactions of parents can range from rejection and anger at being "manipulated" to support and concern.

WHY?

Suicidal behavior is like any other behavior, meaning that it can be negatively or positively reinforced by environmental response. If the motivation for a suicide attempt is to influence a parent to do something (e.g., change his or her mind, pay more attention to the patient) and the attempt succeeds in doing so, then the adolescent learns that suicidal behavior is effective for meeting this need, and therefore may consider making another attempt in the future. Patients with repetitive suicidal behavior may engage in the behavior in order to escape a discordant or unsupportive home environment via hospitalization. Conversely, parents may continue or intensify rejection of the patients as a consequence of the suicidal behavior. Parents may feel that they are being manipulated, or feel that the depressed adolescents should "pull themselves up by their bootstraps." This invalidation may increase the patient's despondency and increase the likelihood of another attempt. Additionally, parental hostility toward an adolescent attempter because of his or her distress and behavior predicts treatment nonattendance. Therefore, the reasons to attend to the environmental response are threefold: it may shed light on the motivation for the suicidal behavior, it may be positively reinforcing suicidal behavior, and it may be a warning sign for nonadherence to treatment.

HOW?

The clinician should assess the environmental response both through direct questioning and observation. Once the clinician has ascertained the motivation for the attempt, he or she can ask the patient the extent to which he or she was successful in achieving those goals. Also, were there any other changes that he or she noticed after the attempt? If so, how might these changes in others' attitudes or behaviors affect a decision about making a suicide attempt in the future? Parallel questions can be asked of the parents. In addition, the clinician can observe the frequency of visits, the nature of interaction between family members, and expressions of concern and/or of hostility on the part of the parents (see Figure 2.11).

CASE EXAMPLE

Joanna was a 14-year-old girl diagnosed with depression. She made a suicide attempt because, according to her, she was trying to get her parents to attend to her requests for help. Joanna's parents felt very guilty and were extremely attentive to her following the attempt. What should the clinician do to further assess the impact of the environmental response on Joanna, and what immediate feedback might the clinician have for the family?

- "To what extent were you successful in achieving your goal [after having asked about motivation for the attempt]?"
- "Do you notice anything different with your family or peers after the attempt?"
- "To what extent do these [responses] make you more [less] likely to attempt suicide in the future?"
- [To parents] "To what extent did the suicide attempt affect your feelings or behavior toward [patient's name]?"

FIGURE 2.11. Environmental response to a suicide attempt.

RESPONSE

The clinician asked Joanna if she has noticed any difference in her parents' behavior, and how that might affect her consideration of a suicide attempt in the future. Joanna responded that "it was almost worth it, because I finally got my parents to pay attention to me." The clinician could suggest to Joanna that perhaps one thing they could work on together is finding ways to get her parents to pay attention to her distress without putting her life on the line. The clinician can then help Joanna communicate this goal to her family prior to discharge.

CASE EXAMPLE

What should the clinician do if Joanna's parents' response in the above-noted case was anger and rejection?

RESPONSE

The clinician should try to get a better picture of what it is about the patient's behavior that the parents find so objectionable. Often, parents and patients benefit from an explanation of the medical model of depression, which helps explain the patient's behavior and feelings without blaming either party.

Domain 2: Psychiatric Disorder

WHAT?

Psychiatric disorders are diseases that affect mood, thoughts, and behavior. Psychiatric disorders have a distinguishable clinical presentation, often run in families, and have a defined course and common causes.

WHY?

Almost all psychiatric disorders are associated with an increased risk for suicidal ideation and behavior. Mood disorders have the strongest association with suicidal ideation and attempt, but this is mostly because they increase the likelihood of suicidal ideation, which in turn increases the risk of an attempt. Restrictive eating disorders and schizophrenia both pose high risks for suicide, but usually this occurs in young adulthood rather than adolescence. Other conditions related to emotional distress (anxiety disorders, especially PTSD) and impulse control (conduct disorder, alcohol and substance abuse), particularly in combination with mood disorder, make it more likely that a person with ideation with a plan will go on to make a suicide attempt.

Among those with a unipolar depressive disorder, mood lability, irritability, and sleep difficulties are associated with an increased risk for suicide attempt or completion. Sleep difficulties are more common and more severe in individuals with mood disorders who attempt or complete suicide, perhaps because sleep-deprived individuals are more irritable and impulsive, and poorer at problem solving. Other indicators of suicidal risk among depressed youth are painful emotions ("I can't stand it") and pathological guilt ("I am a burden to everyone"). Because patients are most likely to complete suicide during their first depressive episode, early diagnosis and treatment are very important.

Young patients with bipolar disorder may have an even higher risk for attempted and completed suicide than those with unipolar disorder. The risk is highest in those with rapid cycling or mixed states, particularly when presenting in a mixed state and in the presence of comorbid alcohol and substance abuse. The mixed state places youth at particularly high risk for suicidal behavior because the patient experiences both the dysphoria and hopelessness of depression and the impulsivity and irritability of mania.

The association between anxiety and suicidal behavior is strongest when the anxiety disorder is comorbid with mood disorder. However, panic disorder, social anxiety disorder, and PTSD appear to increase the risk for suicidal behavior even in the absence of depression. Suicidal behavior is often motivated by a desire to escape the painful emotions associated with anxiety disorders, especially to avoid the negative affect generated by anxiety-provoking situations. Complicated grief (characterized by pining for the deceased, bitterness, and difficulty "letting go") has also been associated with increased levels of suicidal ideation above and beyond other psychopathology.

Impulse control disorders—specifically, conduct disorder and alcohol and substance abuse—make a person with suicidal thoughts more likely to act on those thoughts, probably because of disinhibition and a tendency to take impulsive action. If a gun is available, an intoxicated youth is more likely to use it for a suicide attempt. Alcohol and drug use may also increase depressive affect. Also, youth with these difficulties are more likely to get into legal and disciplinary situations that are themselves precipitants for suicidal behavior. The combination of conduct and substance problems increases suicidal risk more than either condition alone. Patients with bulimia frequently have associated issues with substance abuse and impulsivity, and therefore are at increased risk for suicide attempts because of these characteristics.

HOW?

Every suicidal adolescent should have a careful diagnostic assessment. Although the current severity of symptoms can be assessed using self-report measures, only an interview can help to map the time course of psychiatric disorder and suicidal behavior. We recommend using a time line in which the patient can help the clinician document his or her changes in mood, the course of comorbid difficulties like alcohol abuse or anxiety disorder, and the timing of suicidal ideation and behavior. While knowing that a patient has a given psychiatric condition is important, the role of the clinician at the early assessment stage is to try to find out what aspects of these disorders at a particular point in time make the strongest contribution to the patient's suicidal ideation and behavior.

CASE EXAMPLE

A 15-year-old girl transferred to a new school and shortly thereafter made a suicide attempt. She has a history of depressed mood with passive suicidal ideation since last year but now has also developed symptoms of a social anxiety disorder. How can the clinician determine which condition is of greatest relevance to her suicidal behavior?

RESPONSE

The clinician can plot out the course of her depressive and social anxiety symptoms and note that her suicide attempt came approximately 1 month after the onset of her social anxiety (Figure 2.12).

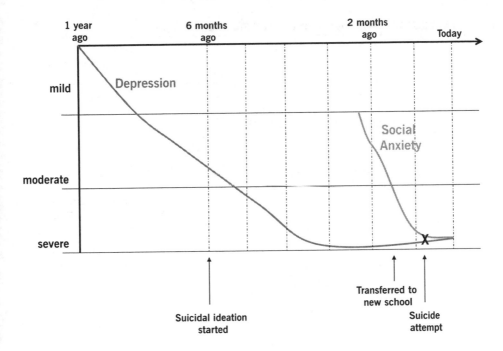

FIGURE 2.12. Sample time line of depression and anxiety symptoms.

Given her depression and anxiety, the clinician asked what made her want to attempt suicide. She responded that the social anxiety at school was so painful that she would rather die than return to a school full of strangers.

Domain 3: Psychological Traits

WHAT?

Certain psychological traits predispose individuals to suicidal behavior. By *traits* we mean characteristic patterns of thinking, feeling, and behaving that are relatively stable, regardless of psychological state. These tendencies may be exacerbated by the presence of depression, but should predate the depressive episode in order to be considered a trait. We describe four important traits to consider with respect to suicidal behavior: (1) hopelessness, (2) lack of ability to access and sustain positive feelings, (3) impulsivity, and (4) emotional dysregulation (see Table 2.3).

TABLE 2.3. Psychological Traits and Suicidal Behavior

	Hopelessness	Lack of access to positive memories	Impulsivity	Impulsive aggression/emotion regulation
Thinking	Negative view of self, future, world	Inability to access and/or sustain positive memories	Don't take in full range of important information for decision making	Tend to view ambiguous situations as dangerous or hostile
Feeling	Sadness, despair, anger	Lack of happiness	Anger	Anger, sadness, irritability; emotional response is big, fast, and long
Acting	Inaction, or high-intent attempt	Act without using previous experience	Act without thinking	Act without thinking in response to provocation or frustration

Hopelessness

WHAT?

Patients who are hopeless are pessimistic about the future, about their own abilities, and about the ability of things to work out. When two people are faced with the same information, the more hopeless person will weight and even distort information so that it will confirm his or her pessimistic worldview, whereas a more optimistic person will weight the same information in such a way as to confirm a more hopeful perspective. A hopeless person is likely to experience negative emotion in response to confirmation of his or her hopeless situation, and consequently either take no action (since it is pointless to even try) or take action that is consistent with a hopeless worldview (such as making a suicide attempt). Sometimes patients are realistically hopeless about a situation—for example, an adolescent who feels trapped in an abusive home situation or bullying at school. In these cases, it is the task of the therapist to help the patient see that these situations can be addressed and take action toward resolving them in collaboration with the patient and relevant adults.

WHY?

Hopelessness is a strong predictor of suicidal ideation, suicide attempts, and suicide completion. Significantly, hopeless individuals are often pessimistic about treatment and therefore drop out. So, hopelessness about treatment must be addressed or the patient may never come back for another appointment.

HOW?

The patient's hopelessness about treatment can be assessed by asking, "On a scale of 1–10, if 1 is really hopeless and 10 is really hopeful, where would you place yourself with regard to being hopeful that we can help you here?" If the patient gives a low number, then the clinician might ask why it isn't lower, what might bring it up, and what might make the person feel even more hopeless. Similar questions can be asked about hopelessness related to other aspects of his or her life circumstances. If the patient has been in treatment before, the clinician should find out what aspects of the treatment the patient found helpful or not helpful. It is understandable that patients may feel hopeless because they did not get better in previous treatment. The therapist might then explain what is different about the proposed treatment, and why the current treatment plan might be more likely to help (without making judgments about the previous therapist or therapy) (see Figure 2.13).

CASE EXAMPLE

A 17-year-old male with chronic depression and suicidal ideation with a plan came for treatment. He reported 2 years of supportive therapy that he says "did not help." When asked how hopeful or hopeless he was about treatment, he rated his hopefulness a 4. How could the therapist respond?

RESPONSE

One response might be "Great, that's a lot more than a 1. Why isn't it lower? And what might make it higher?" The boy went on to say,

---

- "On a scale of 1–10, if 1 is the most hopeless and 10 is the most hopeful about getting better in treatment, where would you place yourself?"
- "Why isn't it lower/higher?"
- "What would make it lower/higher?"
- Follow up with previous experiences in treatment.

FIGURE 2.13. Assessing hopelessness.

"In my previous treatment, the therapist was really nice and listened really well. I talked and talked and after a while I think I ended up feeling worse for talking so much about how bad I felt." The therapist could reply, "It sounds like your previous treatment had a lot of important elements of good care—the therapist was nonjudgmental and a good listener, and you felt safe. We try to do those things here. For many teenagers with depression, that type of treatment is enough, but some, like you, may need more guidance and direction in treatment, in terms of learning different ways of coping with negative emotions that right now are taking over your life. That's the general approach that we take. How does that sound?"

Lack of Ability to Sustain Positive Feelings

WHAT?

Some patients have relative difficulty in experiencing and sustaining positive emotions. This could be the result of a relatively low response to rewarding activities, interference from negative thoughts, or inability to access positive memories.

WHY?

A limited ability to experience positive emotions may contribute to hopelessness, depression, and a decreased ability to identify reasons for living. People under stress will often try to access a positive emotion or a memory of a similar situation in which they successfully dealt with the current challenge. Those who cannot muster or sustain positive emotion have difficulty utilizing such coping approaches. Such individuals may also have difficulty recalling previously learned adaptive ways of coping, which then interferes with their ability to respond effectively to stress. Under stress, a person with this cognitive style has more difficulty comforting him- or herself, and also may be less able to generate a list of appropriate solutions to a given problem and to choose appropriately. All of these difficulties can contribute to suicidal behavior.

HOW?

The clinician should assess the patient's capacity to experience pleasure and determine whether diminished capacity is attributable to a current depressive disorder or is a lifelong pattern. It is better to be as specific as possible, for example, "When is the last time you had a really good time? What did you do? What was fun about it? Are there things you experience that make it difficult for you to enjoy yourself?" To assess the patient's ability to sustain a positive mood, the clinician can ask, "Tell me about the last time you were in a really good mood. How long did it last?" The patient can use a time line to chart his or her mood: how long the positive mood was sustained, the rate at which it decayed, and what feelings and thoughts were related to the decline. To assess the patient's ability to access positive and adaptive memories, the clinician can ask how frequently the patient does so on his or her own, and how stress or negative emotion affects this ability.

Impulsivity and Poor Problem Solving

WHAT?

Impulsivity refers to acting without sufficient forethought. This trait often goes along with poor problem-solving skills, insofar as the person acts before anyone, regardless of intrinsic problem-solving ability, could come up with a viable solution. In addition to impulsivity, many suicide attempters lack the ability to generate a list of viable alternative solutions to problems, to evaluate that list, and to choose a course of action.

WHY?

The majority of adolescent suicide attempts are impulsive. The relationship between impulsivity and problem solving is bidirectional. Impulsive action short-circuits problem solving. Conversely, the lack of ability to generate a list of viable solutions also predisposes the suicide attempter to impulsive action. Both sets of difficulties are frequently found in adolescent suicide attempters—impulsivity and difficulty in generating and selecting appropriate solutions to problems.

HOW?

To assess the trait of impulsivity, the clinician can ask, "Do you often act without thinking? Could you give me an example of that? Would you say that is typical of you?" The clinician can also return to the suicide attempt and ask what happened between the time the patient first thought about suicide and the time he or she made the attempt. The clinician can also assess problem solving by asking, "What other alternatives did you consider at that time? What about now? Do you find that coming up with a list of solutions to a problem is harder for you under stress?"

Emotion Dysregulation

WHAT?

Emotion dysregulation, the broad category under which impulsive aggression falls, refers to emotional responses to a given situation that differ from the average. This includes the threshold for responding (i.e., it takes something relatively small to set off an emotional reaction), amplitude (i.e., greater intensity of the emotional response), and duration (i.e., longer response than expected). For example, if a person without a vulnerability to emotion dysregulation gets a parking ticket, he or she might feel mildly upset, pay the fine, and move on. A person with emotion dysregulation might lose his or her temper with the police officer (lower threshold for emotional responding and greater intensity) and remain upset about the ticket several days later (longer duration). *Impulsive aggression* is the tendency to respond to provocation or frustration with hostility or aggression. Impulsive aggression, sometimes termed *reactive aggression,* is different from an aggressive act that the individual plans (sometimes referred to as instrumental aggression).

WHY?

A precipitant may elicit a "dysregulated" emotional response, which in turn makes it impossible for the youth to generate viable alternatives or otherwise access his or her skill set to deal with an emotionally challenging situation. Chronic depression, bipolar disorder, sleep deprivation, and alcohol/substance abuse can all contribute to greater emotion dysregulation. It is important, though, to distinguish between temporary impairment in emotion regulation due to disease, sleep deprivation, or substance abuse as opposed to emotion dysregulation as a lifelong personality trait.

Especially in adolescent and young adult suicide completers and attempters, impulsive aggression, above and beyond depression, contributes to suicidal risk. Patients with impulsive aggression will frequently interpret ambiguous situations as hostile and respond in kind, thus generating conflict unnecessarily. Some of these conflictual situations can be a precipitant for a suicide attempt. In addition, such patients become emotionally dysregulated in response to perceived hostility, and are therefore less likely to use rational problem solving. One reason why children of parents who attempt suicide are more likely to attempt it themselves is that impulsive aggression runs in families. As this trait passes from parent to child, the risk for suicidal behavior is also transmitted. Brain imaging, postmortem studies of brain material of suicide completers, and other types of biological studies have shown that biological changes associated with suicidal behavior and impulsive aggression are very similar. Therefore homocidal ideation should also be assessed in suicidal patients.

HOW?

Often, the degree of emotion dysregulation or tendency to impulsive aggression can be ascertained from the description of the suicide attempt. Then, the clinician can determine if this is indeed a lifelong pattern for the patient or something out of the ordinary. Suggested questions for assessing emotion dysregulation and impulsive aggression are found in Figure 2.14.

CASE EXAMPLE

Six months ago, Joe, a 16-year-old male, made a serious suicide attempt. At that time, he began receiving traditional CBT for his depression. He appeared to be making good progress, with a significant decrease in his depressive symptoms. But 5 weeks into treatment, after a fight with his girlfriend, Joe cut both his wrists with a razor and required medical attention. How can we conceptualize this behavior?

RESPONSE

The clinician may have believed that treating Joe's depression protected him from a reattempt because he could use the skills learned in CBT. However, it is likely that Joe had difficulty with impulsive aggression that was not apparent when he was not under stress. The clinician refocused treatment on learning emotion regulation skills so that under stress, he could remain calm enough to use the skills he had learned.

- "Would you say that your mood is even, or more up and down?"
- "Can you tell me what things have led to your mood changing a lot recently?"
- "How upset did you get, and how long did you stay upset?"
- "When you are upset, to what extent are you able to problem-solve or calm yourself down?"
- "When you are upset, how likely are you to do something rash, and if so, what?"

FIGURE 2.14. Assessing emotion regulation and impulsive aggression.

Domain 4: Family/Environmental Stressors and Supports

WHAT?

The most common family and environmental contributors to suicidal risk are parent–child discord, parental psychiatric illness, maltreatment, bullying at school, and same-sex attraction. Often, these stressors are interrelated. Parent–child discord is more likely to occur if a parent is depressed and irritable, and parental psychiatric disorder also increases the likelihood of child maltreatment. Youth with same-sex attraction are often bullied and rejected at school and at home.

WHY?

Parent–child discord is the most common precipitant for suicidal behavior in younger adolescents. This does not mean that the fighting between parent and child caused the attempt, because there are many other households where the same level of discord does not lead to suicidal behavior. However, family conflict is a contributing factor to suicidal behavior in a vulnerable adolescent. Discord at home also makes an adolescent less likely to recover from depression, and more likely to relapse.

Conversely, family and environmental characteristics can also protect against risk for suicidal behavior, even when patients have other conditions that make suicidal behavior more likely, such as depression. These characteristics include a patient's having a positive and confiding relationship with at least one parent; family members' doing things together (such as eating meals and spending leisure time together); and evidence of active parental monitoring and supervision of the adolescent's activities. Involvement in prosocial activities and peer groups, and having a positive connection with school, are also protective.

Parental psychiatric disorders predispose children to suicidal risk in two ways. First, because psychiatric disorders and suicidal behavior are familial, the offspring of such parents are at increased risk for depression and suicidal behavior. Second, current depression in parents is associated with increased distress and symptoms in children, and when children are in treatment for depression it interferes with their successful recovery. Most important, treatment of maternal depression has been shown to improve treatment outcome in children. Therefore, assessment and referral for parental psychiatric disorder is very important to ensure a full recovery for the child.

A history of maltreatment—namely, neglect or physical or sexual abuse—greatly increases the risk for a suicide attempt in several ways.

Maltreatment increases the risk for depression and also for PTSD, both of which make suicidal behavior more likely. In addition, youth with a history of abuse are more likely to have high levels of impulsive aggression, and, when confronted with an ambiguous social situation, tend to interpret neutral situations as hostile. Current abuse is an emergency that calls for removal of the child from the home. Bullying is also an important contributor to suicidal risk, and can be thought of as abuse by peers. Same-sex attraction, even if the adolescent has not acted on it, greatly increases the risk for suicide attempt, depression, and substance abuse. Most commonly, youth with same-sex attraction are targeted by bullies at school, experience rejection at home, and are vulnerable to sexual exploitation because of a real or perceived lack of social support. In addition, especially for youth raised in households in which homosexuality is viewed negatively, the experience of same-sex attraction can be a source of great distress. On the other hand, just as bullying and peer rejection can increase suicidal risk, having a sense of connection with friends and with school and being involved in school activities can be protective, even in the presence of other risk factors for suicidal behavior.

HOW?

Figure 2.15 lists some sample questions for assessing common environmental stressors and supports. The precipitants and motivations for the suicide attempt may also provide some clues as to sources of stress for the patient. Parents may be resistant to focusing on their own problems, and the clinician needs to use his or her own judgment about whether to broach this issue at the initial meeting or wait until after a relationship has been established. The routine use of a brief screening questionnaire for parental depression can provide an entrée to such a discussion. The clinician can explain that parental recovery will greatly enhance the chances that the child will get better. If the patient discloses abuse, and it is ongoing, most local regulations require that this be reported. Additionally, the clinician must determine if it is safe for the patient to return home. Past abuse also may need to be reported, depending on local reporting requirements and the current risk to the patient and others. Bullying is not necessarily an emergency, but most schools have antibullying policies. The clinician should work with the patient and family to make sure that the school policy is properly implemented and reflects the needs of the patient.

Asking about same-sex attraction can feel awkward, both for the clinician and for the patient. Ideally, this should be assessed in a mat-

- Parent–child relationship
  "How do you get along with your parents?"
  "How often do you fight and about what?"
  "What do your parents criticize you about?"
  "How do your parents show their support of you?"
  "What things do you do together?"
  "Do they usually know what you are doing?"

- Parental mental health
  [Ask parent] "Have you even had a sad mood for at least 2 weeks with difficulty functioning?" Or ask parent to fill out the Center for Epidemiologic Studies Depression Scale (CES-D). Also ask about anxiety and substance use.

- Abuse and family violence
  "Has anyone ever hit you repeatedly or threatened you physically?"
  "Has anyone touched you in a sexual way without your permission?"
  "Do you fear for your safety at home?"
  "Have you seen physical fights at home?"
  "Are you afraid for the safety of any family members?"

- School
  "How do you like school?"
  "What sort of connection do you have with school, the kids there, and the teachers?"
  "Is there any one teacher that you feel especially connected with?"

- Peers
  "Do you feel connected to a group of friends?"
  "What sort of things do you do together? Are you involved in any kind of clubs or organized activities together?"
  "Do your friends tend to get in trouble or use drugs and alcohol?"

- Bullying
  "Have you ever been repeatedly teased or hassled at school?"
  "Do you feel like you don't belong in the school you go to?"

- Sexual orientation
  "Would you say that you are mainly attracted to boys, girls, or both?"

FIGURE 2.15. Assessing environmental stressors and supports.

ter-of-fact way. It may be helpful to preface questions about sexual history as follows: "I would like to ask you some questions related to sexual thoughts and behavior. I know it might be a little awkward, but it is an important part of life, as important as the other things we have been talking about. Would that be okay with you? What we talk about, like everything else, stays in here between us, unless you are talking about a situation in which your life is in danger." If the patient declines, then the clinician can simply say, "Maybe we can return to this when you are feeling more comfortable about it."

CASE EXAMPLE

During the initial interview with a 15-year-old girl and her mother, the mother appears to be quite sad. The patient's mother has also endorsed many current depressive symptoms on a self-report screening questionnaire. What should the clinician do next?

RESPONSE

The clinician should ask to speak with the mother in private and share with her the observation that her score on the questionnaire suggests she may be depressed. The clinician may ask for her reaction to this information. If the mother says she would prefer not to talk about it, then the clinician should indicate that he or she respects the mother's privacy. The clinician can go on to explain that the reason for the screening is that depression often runs in families and that depression in a parent may make it harder for the treatment of the child to work. The clinician can offer the mother the open invitation to revisit the issue, and can provide a number where he or she can be reached for a confidential conversation in the event that the mother changes her mind.

Domain 5: Availability of Lethal Methods

WHAT?

Lethal methods are those methods of suicide associated with a high fatality rate, such as guns, medications, and household chemicals.

WHY?

Suicidal behavior in adolescence is often impulsive, and the availability of a lethal method can make the difference between a low-intent suicide attempt and death. Around 10% of adolescents who kill themselves have no evidence of a psychiatric disorder, and up to 40% of adolescents under the age of 16 who kill themselves display no evidence of a psychiatric disorder. The only difference between youth who have no clear disorder who kill themselves and healthy living controls is the presence of a loaded gun or other lethal method in the home. Many studies have shown that the proximity and availability of lethal methods (including acetaminophen tablets, pesticides, and toxic fumes from heating gas

- Suicide by firearms is the most common method of completed suicide in both adolescent girls and boys.
- Suicide completers are 4–10 times more likely to have a gun in their home than similar controls.
- Youth who completed suicide but did not have a clear psychiatric disorder were 31 times more likely to have a loaded gun in the home than were similar living controls.
- Even guns that are locked pose some risk for suicide, although securing guns is better than leaving them loaded.

FIGURE 2.16. Facts for families on firearms and suicide.

or automobiles) have a big influence on the suicide rate, especially in adolescents and young adults. Since guns are the most common method of completed suicide in the United States, we focus on the assessment of availability and storage of guns, and provide some facts for families in Figure 2.16.

HOW?

The clinician should inquire about the availability and storage of guns, medication, household chemicals, and knives, and should then make recommendations for removal or safe storage. However, the clinician should not assume that just because he or she has discussed the importance of removing lethal means with the family they will remove guns from the home. Many individuals keep guns at home for protection; for them, removal is tantamount to putting their family members at risk, despite evidence that for every justifiable homicide there are many suicides related to having a gun in the home. In one study, we found that only one in four parents who said they would remove a gun from the home actually did so. Those most likely to remove guns were single parents, probably because when we were speaking with the mothers, we were speaking directly with the gun owners. On the other hand, those least likely to remove guns were married, and in discordant relationships with a spouse who had difficulty with alcohol or drug abuse. If the gun owner was a substance-abusing husband with whom the wife had a discordant relationship, it is understandable why she was reluctant to pursue this line of conversation with her husband. Therefore, it is important to speak directly to the gun owner about safety issues (see

- "Are there guns at home?"
- [If so] "What kind? How are they stored?"
- "Who owns them?"
- Then ask these questions of the gun owner:
  - "Why do you have them?"
  - "Would you be willing to consider removing them from the home during this period of time?"
  - "If not, would you be willing to secure them?"

FIGURE 2.17. How to negotiate about removing guns from the homes of suicidal youth.

Figure 2.17). Furthermore, the clinician must be willing to accept less than perfect solutions at times—such as securing the firearms instead of removing them.

ASSESSING IMMINENT SUICIDAL RISK

In the preceding section, we have described assessment domains that inform a comprehensive treatment plan for depressed and suicidal youth. A certain subset of characteristics from these assessment domains (described below) will help determine imminent suicidal risk, and also help determine level of care. More intensive treatment, such as inpatient or partial hospitalization, is indicated when (1) the patient cannot adhere to a safety plan and is in danger at a lower intensity of treatment; (2) the patient has not made progress at a lower level of care; or (3) level of functioning is such that outpatient care is insufficient (e.g., a patient who is too anxious and depressed to attend school).

An individual is at acute or imminent suicidal risk if he or she cannot adhere to a safety plan, or is clinically regarded as highly unlikely to do so. A *safety plan* (see Chapter 4 for more detail) is a set of strategies developed collaboratively among the clinician, patient, and parents that outlines how the patient and family will cope with recurrent suicidal thoughts and urges. Below we examine the proximal risk factors that make it unlikely a patient can adhere to a safety plan. We use the following mnemonic to determine risk: *AID ILL SAD DADS*. In this mnemonic, *AID* and *ILL* refer to proximal risk factors, and *SAD* and *DADS* to distal risk factors.

Proximal Risk Factors

Proximal risk factors for suicidal behavior are those factors related to current clinical state and social context that interfere with the person's ability to adhere to a safety plan. Such risk factors interfere with safety either by diminishing the ability to cope or exacerbating the intensity of suicidal urges.

- Agitation. This is a state of acute discomfort, arousal, and restlessness, characterized by insomnia, anxiety (especially panic disorder or PTSD), agitated depression, or drug-induced restlessness. The patient is driven to consider suicide because he or she wants to escape this state of acute discomfort and distress.
- Intent. Individuals who want to die are at highest risk for an attempt or completed suicide. They frequently are hopeless about the future, have suicidal ideation with a plan, and if they have already made an attempt, regret having survived.
- Despair. Despair is the experience of feeling extremely sad to the point where it is painful and intolerable. As in those with agitation, the motivation of suicidal individuals is to escape the suffering associated with the painful depression. This is a very dangerous indicator in those with limited ability to tolerate distress or regulate painful emotions.
- Instability. A patient whose mood, judgment, or commitment to avoid resorting to suicide fluctuates widely as a consequence of brain injury, the mood lability of unipolar depression or mixed or rapid cycling bipolar disorder, imminent substance use, a high level of impulsive aggression, or psychosis is unlikely to be able to adhere to a safety plan.
- Loss. The loss of a relationship or role (e.g., loss of a job or important position like captain of the football team), or of health or function, often is an acute precipitant for suicidal ideation and behavior across the lifespan.
- Lethal method. The ready availability of a gun or other lethal means of suicide increases the likelihood of a fatal suicide attempt.

Distal Risk Factors

More distal risk factors for suicidal behavior are important in treatment planning, but not as important in assessing imminent risk. Such risk factors can be remembered as follows:

- **S**uicide history, both a personal and a family history of suicidal behavior. *The more recent the attempt, the higher the risk, with the highest risk for reattempt within the first 3 months after the initial attempt, especially if the patient has continued suicidal ideation and depression.* Additionally, having both a personal and family history of suicidal behavior increases the risk for suicidal behavior. However, a positive personal and/or family history does not convey any information about the timing of the risk.
- **A**nhedonia. The inability to experience or sustain positive feelings predisposes a person to ongoing depression and suicidal ideation but does not convey imminent risk.
- **D**ifficult course. Patients who have been tried on a variety of medications, psychotherapies, and programs without experiencing relief begin to despair of ever recovering. *If the patient then becomes acutely hopeless about his or her future and about treatment, this would lead to an increase in imminent risk.*
- **D**ifficult treatment history. Patients who have a history of being nonadherent with their treatment regimens, changing providers frequently, and/or having difficulty engaging with treatment providers may similarly become hopeless about treatment working, leading to increased risk.
- **A**buse and trauma. A history of abuse and exposure to other types of violence increases the risk for suicidal behavior—but not at any particular point in time. A person with a history of abuse may be more difficult to engage, may have symptoms of PTSD, and may have more chronic difficulties with self-esteem, all of which have therapeutic implications. However, *a patient who is currently in an abusive situation and feels trapped is at markedly elevated risk for engaging in a suicide attempt to escape what may be perceived as an impossible social situation.*
- **D**isconnection. Patients who are socially isolated (not involved with peers, family, school, or work) are at extremely high risk of completing suicide. However, disconnection does not convey imminent risk unless a major source of support has suddenly departed from the patient's social network (e.g., best friend moved across the country).
- **S**ubstance abuse. Alcohol and drug abuse increases the risk for completed and attempted suicide, but only intoxication increases imminent risk. Moreover, in adolescents and in adults, those who have difficulties with alcohol or other substances are much more sensitive to stressful life events such as loss of a relationship or a job.

CASE EXAMPLE

An adolescent boy presents in the emergency room with self-cutting behavior, suicidal ideation with a plan and intent, intoxication with alcohol, and bipolar disorder with a mixed state. This patient shows difficulty with emotion regulation (self-cutting behavior), and is emotionally labile due both to his substance abuse and his bipolar disorder. Is this patient at imminent risk for suicide? If so, why?

RESPONSE

The patient is at very high risk for suicidal behavior because he is clinically unstable and at the same time shows high intent. Ideally, this patient should be hospitalized, his bipolar disorder stabilized, and a referral made to manage his bipolar disorder and alcohol use.

DISPOSITION

On the basis of this risk assessment, the clinician needs to make a determination about the required intensity of mental health services. Patients who are highly suicidal, who are not regretful about having made an attempt, who have shown high suicidal intent, or who are too unstable to be able to make and adhere to a safety plan should be hospitalized for their own safety. If the family objects, it is usually better to try a modified treatment plan that the family can adhere to, such as going to a day hospital or to intensive outpatient treatment. No existing data support the efficacy of hospitalization for the management of suicidal behavior, so it is important for the clinician not to be too rigid. It is important to have a clear plan for a transition from inpatient to outpatient settings, since it is during this transition that the completed and attempted suicide rate is the highest. We recommend that the clinician who is going to be seeing the patient on an outpatient basis meet the patient and family prior to discharge whenever possible, as there are data to indicate that this will increase adherence to the first appointment, which should be offered as close as possible to the date of discharge.

CASE EXAMPLE

An adolescent boy who did relatively well in treatment presented with a recurrence of suicidal ideation with a plan and increased depressive symptoms, despite continued adherence to medication and psychotherapy. When the clinician asked if anything had changed, he confided that he had become increasingly aware of his same-sex attraction and was very distressed about it. The clinician and the patient reviewed his safety plan, and despite his ideation, he indicated that he could use his coping skills to manage the ideation. An additional follow-up appointment was scheduled that week. Was this patient at high imminent suicidal risk? Why or why not?

RESPONSE

Although this patient presented with suicidal ideation with a plan, it was in the context of a strong therapeutic relationship with the therapist and a track record of being able to adhere to and implement a safety plan. Moreover, there was a clear precipitant. A higher level of care may have been disruptive to the functional working relationship between therapist and patient.

CASE EXAMPLE

A teenage boy with dysthymic disorder, conduct disorder, and substance abuse who was at the beginning stages of treatment and in the midst of a fight with his mother threatened to kill himself. He had not previously been suicidal. The mother called, panicked, and wanted to know if she should bring her son to the emergency room for an evaluation. Was this patient at imminent risk for suicidal behavior?

RESPONSE

The comorbidity pattern of conduct disorder, substance abuse, and mood disorder in an adolescent male is a common one seen in completed suicide. Nevertheless, it is unclear if the threat that the patient was making reflected intent to die or was simply said in anger. The therapist asked to speak with the patient; in this case, he admitted that he had not had suicidal ideation, did not intend to make a suicide attempt, and had only made this statement in anger. The therapist explained to the patient how statements like his should be taken seriously, but that he should only use such language if it really reflected his feelings. An appointment was scheduled for the next day in order to reassess the patient, confirm initial impressions, and provide additional psychoeducation about suicidal threats and behavior to patient and mother.

KEY POINTS

- Five key domains of suicidal behavior to assess in order to determine risk and formulate an appropriate treatment plan:

    1. Characteristics of current and past suicidal ideation and behavior.

    2. Psychiatric disorder.

    3. Psychological traits.

    4. Family/environmental stressors.

    5. Availability of lethal methods.

- Inpatient or partial hospitalization is indicated in the event of any of the following:

    1. The patient cannot adhere to a safety plan and is in danger at a lower intensity of treatment.

    2. The patient has not made progress at a lower level of care.

    3. Level of functioning is such that outpatient care is insufficient (e.g., a patient who is too anxious and depressed to attend school.

CHAPTER 3

Important Components of Effective Treatment

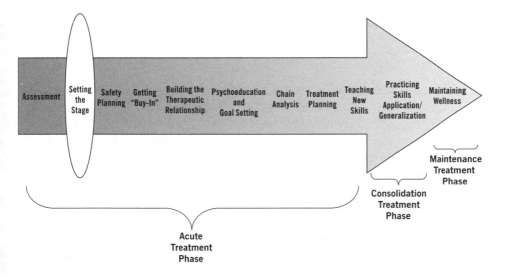

WHAT YOU WILL LEARN IN THIS CHAPTER

- The critical elements needed to effectively treat suicidal and depressed adolescents:
  - The importance of the treatment team.
  - The functions of supervision.
  - Guidelines for establishing 24-hour coverage.
  - What to do if you do not have a team.
- Helpful therapist characteristics.
- The nature of the therapeutic relationship.

85

In this chapter, we discuss the critical elements a therapist needs in order to effectively treat suicidal and depressed adolescents. As depicted in Figure 3.1, these components include (1) the organizational environment; (2) the individual as therapist; and ultimately (3) the therapeutic relationship between the therapist and the teen.

THE ORGANIZATIONAL ENVIRONMENT

The optimal organizational environment for treating suicidal teens promotes a team approach, provides regular supervision and consultation, devotes attention and resources to the assurance of continuity of care, and has 24-hour backup available.

The Team Approach

Treatment of suicidal and depressed teens presents multiple challenges for the therapist. The cornerstone of the clinic culture we espouse is a team approach to treatment that allows for shared decision making and provides a supportive environment for the therapist working with this challenging population.

The treatment team is multidisciplinary, and is comprised of therapists, nurse clinicians (who may also conduct psychotherapy), and child psychiatrists. This structure allows for the provision of comprehensive services for our patients. As discussed in the introduction, our treatment team at the STAR Clinic adheres to a medical model of psychiatric illness, whereby depression and comorbid psychiatric conditions

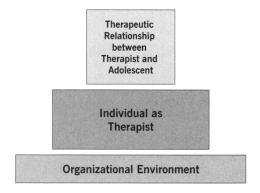

FIGURE 3.1. Framework for conducting treatment with depressed and suicidal adolescents: the three layers.

are viewed as biologically based brain disorders. Thus, throughout the book we refer to the adolescent as the *patient*. We appreciate that some therapists prefer the term *client* as a means of highlighting the collaborative nature of the relationship. We also agree with this terminology, and while we refer to adolescents as *patients*, we treat them as *clients*. Our multidisciplinary approach also facilitates the management of the multiple additional medical and psychosocial difficulties that commonly accompany depression and suicidality in adolescents.

Clinicians working with this population are frequently required to make decisions about imminent risk and appropriate level of care. Such clinical decisions can be complicated and anxiety-provoking, and we feel that no provider, no matter how experienced, should have to face these decisions alone. Rather, consultation from a team of expert clinicians maximizes our ability to monitor for safety.

Incorporating the varied perspectives of team members also optimizes the process of case conceptualization. In the STAR Clinic, this occurs during weekly treatment team meetings attended by all team members, during which we review cases. Team members share clinical formulations and encourage one another to consider alternative approaches. Within the treatment team meeting, we review an individualized treatment plan for each adolescent that incorporates a range of interventions including medications, psychotherapy (individual and/or family), case management, and school consultation. In the multidisciplinary setting of the treatment team meeting, case conceptualization is informed by feedback from each discipline.

Supervision

Providing treatment for suicidal and depressed teens can be demanding. Even the best of therapists needs ongoing supervision, in addition to the weekly treatment team meeting. STAR Clinic therapists attend individual supervision weekly, with a focus on three essential components: enhancing the therapist's skill set, optimizing use of the therapist's own personal characteristics, and providing support and encouragement (see Figure 3.2).

Supervision focuses primarily on enhancing the therapist's skill set and fine-tuning the delivery of treatment. We find that frequent review of videotaped sessions is uniquely informative during the process of case conceptualization and treatment planning. Videotaping bypasses the therapist's subjective recall of the events of a session and can help identify important elements of a case conceptualization that may not have initially been apparent to the therapist. For example, a therapist

> • Enhance the therapist's skill set.
> • Optimize the therapist's use of his or her own personal characteristics.
> • Provide support and encouragement.

FIGURE 3.2. Main components of supervision.

may have initially conceptualized a case based on a deficit in distress tolerance skills, but upon tape review, the teen's hopelessness becomes an additional important area for focused intervention. The videotape review also captures both patient and therapist nonverbal behavior that may be important topics for supervision. The pace and timing of interventions is readily apparent during videotape review, which can increase awareness and allow for fine-tuning of these elements of treatment.

One-on-one supervision that includes a review of videotaped sessions also provides the unique opportunity to identify the ways in which the therapist's own characteristics contribute to the therapeutic process. While watching videotaped sessions, the therapist can observe how his or her interaction with the teen affects the course of the session. For example, a videotape may reveal that the therapist showed facial expressions of discomfort or disapproval that led the adolescent to avoid further discussion of the topic. During supervision, we encourage therapists to discuss their own emotional reactions to the teen and to the therapeutic process. It is especially important to discuss instances where the therapist's own feelings or reactions may be limiting his or her ability to engage optimally in the therapeutic process.

CASE EXAMPLE

Anna was a 15-year-old patient who had attempted suicide 4 weeks ago by overdose. Anna was stabilized medically, transferred to the inpatient psychiatric unit, and released after 4 days. She subsequently attended a partial hospitalization program for 3 weeks. One of us worked with Anna on an outpatient basis, and another provided individual supervision. Anna's suicide attempt indicated very high intent (i.e., she planned her suicide for several weeks, wrote a suicide note, and took the pills when nobody was home and there was little chance of anyone discovering her) and high lethality (i.e., she took approximately 100 tablets of acetaminophen [Tylenol]). Furthermore, she expressed intense disappointment that "it did not work"—her mother unexpectedly came home and discovered her. Anna's father, with whom she had enjoyed a very close relationship, had died from suicide several years before. Anna's present family situation was chaotic and conflictual. The motivation for her attempt was to "be with my dad and escape the pain of life." Although Anna agreed to adhere to a safety plan, she continued to endorse high-intensity suicidal ideation coupled with regret that she had not died. Furthermore, she had difficulty identifying reasons for living, and felt strongly that she would ultimately die from suicide, even if not imminently.

During tape review, both therapist and supervisor recognized that the therapist appeared to be uncharacteristically conservative in session regarding her expectations for Anna. Despite what appeared to be a solid therapeutic alliance, the therapist was hesitant regarding moving Anna toward change. During supervision, therapist and supervisor together identified and discussed how the therapist's own fear regarding Anna's safety was affecting the therapeutic process. First and foremost, the supervisor validated the therapist's concerns—Anna certainly exhibited multiple factors indicative of very high risk for suicide. The supervisor encouraged the therapist to consider how she might balance validating Anna's difficult life circumstances while also avoiding becoming overwhelmed along with Anna. It became evident that the therapist needed to push for change in order to help Anna commit to living and to treatment. These discussions helped to identify the therapist's tentativeness, validated the therapist's worries about the patient, and provided the impetus to try a more assertive stance with Anna.

For this case, let us imagine the outcome if the therapist were treating Anna *without* supervision. First and foremost, she may have been less aware of how her own fear that Anna would kill herself was affecting treatment. She may have relied strictly on validation of Anna's difficult life situation, without concurrently working toward helping Anna to identify the things in her life that she could control. Without encouragement from her supervisor to gently push Anna, it is understandable that the therapist may have become paralyzed by fear and hopelessness along with Anna. The likely result would have been an inability to move forward and collaborate on a treatment plan.

In our view, the practice of limiting the number of actively suicidal patients on a therapist's caseload, although necessary, is not sufficient to successfully manage these difficult patients. It certainly takes a team, either through consultation or shared management, to effectively manage suicidal patients. The challenging nature of providing treatment for suicidal and depressed teens requires that therapists receive ongoing support and encouragement. Supervision can help the therapist retain perspective about the teen's overall progress toward goals while also attending to the immediate details of treatment. Additionally, the supervisor and therapist should be mindful of each individual therapist's limits regarding appropriate caseload, with particular attention to the number of patients on a therapist's caseload who are in the acute phase of treatment.

Attention to Continuity of Care

The risk of suicide is highest during transitions in care—particularly when a patient is moving from a more intense level of care, such as inpatient hospitalization, to outpatient care. Contributors to this increased risk include the following: a return to stressors similar to those that resulted in the hospitalization, lack of coordination between inpatient and outpatient teams, and barriers for the patient and family regarding follow-through with the recommended discharge plans. We therefore take steps to ensure continuity of care and adherence to referral, particularly when a patient moves from one level of care to another. We routinely meet with a representative from other programs in our department that refer to us in order to discuss shared patients and potential referrals. When newly referred patients are still at a higher level of care, we make arrangements to meet the patient and family there *before* their appointment in our program. This practice has been shown to improve adherence, likely because the patient and family have a chance to meet the clinician and begin to build rapport. Additionally, the therapist can take this opportunity to address any patient and family concerns about the transition of care. This strategy helps to ease the transition from one service provider to another. More concretely, but just as important, we offer an initial appointment shortly after discharge from the other program.

Twenty-Four-Hour Backup

Therapists who treat suicidal patients must be able to provide 24-hour backup, preferably by having access to a local psychiatric emergency room and inpatient hospital. Some communities also have 24-hour psychiatric mobile crisis teams that travel to the patient's home in attempt to diffuse a crisis, assess risk, and/or divert hospitalization. We routinely include the phone numbers of the local emergency rooms and crisis teams with our personal contact information; we encourage these services to contact us to consult about a disposition for our patients in crisis. This is an essential element of the safety plan, described in Chapter 4, and the therapist should discuss with the patient and family specifics regarding when and how to access these services. Dialogue between the therapist and the providers of emergency services is helpful in order to preserve continuity of care and fidelity to the treatment plan.

While we do make ourselves available after hours to emergency providers, we do not routinely provide our own home and/or cell phone numbers to patients. Our rationale for this recommendation is threefold. First, treating suicidal teens is a demanding and intense profession. We believe therapists need to have time and space away from the work environment in order to take care of themselves. For therapists who treat high-risk patients, it is essential to have protected time during which one can recharge, maintain one's own personal life, and avoid burnout. Second, many of our patients have limited exposure to adults who effectively maintain their own personal boundaries. Therefore, we encourage therapists to model respect for their own boundaries in this way. Third, we aim to send the message to our patients that we are working collaboratively to equip them with the skills they need to solve their own problems ("I want to empower you to be your own therapist, so you can handle whatever comes your way in life"). As such, we encourage self-reliance and independence so that our patients develop a sense of self-efficacy.

Building a Team

We appreciate that not all therapists work within a setting where a treatment team exists. Although we believe a treatment team approach is ideal for working with suicidal youth, we know this is not always possible. If the therapist does not have access to a treatment team, we recommend that he or she develop a professional network for supervision and ongoing consultation. This network may include other therapists, clinicians, and psychiatrists in the community who are treating similar patients. When face-to-face meetings are not possible, such supervision and consultation can also occur via phone or videoconferencing.

THE INDIVIDUAL AS THERAPIST

When conducting treatment, a therapist draws from two categories of skills—technical skills and interpersonal skills. The effective therapist fluidly incorporates and integrates both sets of skills. We describe these as skills rather than qualities because we believe that both technical and interpersonal skills can be studied, learned, and improved upon with supervision and increased self-awareness.

Technical Skills

Technical skills include skills in assessment, as well as skills in therapy-specific techniques. We have already introduced the key skills required to assess and monitor depression and suicidal risk in Chapters 1 and 2. Therapy-specific techniques include provision of support and encouragement, cognitive restructuring, emotion regulation, problem solving, and family interventions. The implementation of these techniques is the focus of the remainder of this book.

In order to work effectively with suicidal teens in the treatment model described in this book, we recommend that therapists have a minimum of a master's-level degree in a mental-health-related field. Additionally, the therapist should have basic knowledge of adolescent development as well as clinical experience in CBT and family treatment. Often, these therapy-specific techniques are the focus of our professional training and ongoing supervision. Since new information is frequently available, it is also expected that therapists will continue to expand their repertoire of technical skills throughout their careers. We do not mean to imply that CBT is the only psychotherapeutic approach that will be helpful with depressed and suicidal teens. However, most of the empirical work in the field has focused on CBT, and it is the basis of our treatment work as well. Since our therapeutic orientation is based in CBT, this is the type of treatment we emphasize in this book.

As we have also discussed previously, review of videotaped sessions is a good way to assess the quality of specific therapeutic techniques and technical skills. Role play with a supervisor can be a way to rehearse, improve, and consolidate therapeutic approaches to specific patients. If the supervisee is anticipating problems in implementing a particular technique, the supervisor can invite the therapist to play the role of the patient, so that the supervisor can model possible approaches.

Interpersonal Skills

Good treatment relies not only on a therapist's technical skill set but also on his or her own interpersonal skills. These interpersonal skills include the ability to collaborate, defer judgment, and project self-confidence, as well as assertiveness, flexibility, and appropriate "use of self" (see also Figure 3.3). While these qualities come more naturally to some than

- Be willing and able to collaborate.
- Bring a nonjudgmental presence.
- Communicate self-confidence.
- Demonstrate assertiveness.
- Be flexible.
- Incorporate appropriate "use of self."

FIGURE 3.3. Interpersonal skills helpful in the treatment of depressed and suicidal adolescents.

to others, we want to emphasize strongly that *all* of these interpersonal skills can be learned and enhanced. With awareness and willingness, therapists can improve these interpersonal skills through supervision and clinical experience.

First and foremost, the therapist must work collaboratively as a partner in treatment with the adolescent. While this collaborative approach is a basic element of CBT, it is particularly important in working with adolescents because of their developmental needs. The main developmental task of adolescence is to make a transition toward greater autonomy and responsibility. Therefore, a collaborative treatment model that encourages the teen to take an active role in his or her own treatment is developmentally appropriate. Most teens find this approach to be refreshing, because most often the adult–teen relationship outside the home that they are used to is that of teacher and student—a relationship that is necessarily hierarchical. Also, adolescents' experiences with other healthcare providers may not have allowed for much input from the teen; frequently healthcare providers bypass adolescents and coordinate services primarily with the parent. This can lead adolescents to feel disempowered, and to regard the treatment provider as an agent for their parents, rather than someone working to address their own needs. For treatment to succeed, it is important for the adolescent to feel that he or she has a say in the direction of treatment. In essence, in order for the treatment to be successful, the adolescent has to "own" the treatment. This is only possible if he or she has substantial input into the goals and methods of therapy, not only at the outset, but throughout treatment.

Perhaps more so than with any other clinical population, the therapist needs to bring a nonjudgmental presence to the treatment of adolescents. Maintaining a nonjudgmental approach does *not* imply approval or agreement. *Rather, a nonjudgmental approach is based on the premise that every behavior or choice serves a valid purpose and originates from a valid need.* The therapist aims to help the patient see that there are other ways to behave and function that can more effectively meet the same need. Linehan (1993) has effectively articulated the dialectic between the need for a patient to be accepted and also the need for a patient to change. It is very difficult for a patient to have the strength to tackle difficult behaviors if he or she does not feel validated. Additionally, if adolescents feel the therapist is judging them, then they will be less likely to disclose. Therefore a nonjudgmental presence helps create the environment necessary for change.

A nonjudgmental approach is particularly applicable for working with adolescents, given that a central developmental task of adolescence is the development of self-identity. During this developmental process, experimentation with various expressions of the self is necessary. Teens often experience adults as being particularly judgmental of their means of self-expression (e.g., hairstyle, clothing, piercing, tattoos). Therefore, it is essential to strive to create a safe, accepting therapeutic environment in which the adolescent can comfortably explore these aspects of self-expression.

PATIENT: You haven't said anything about my tongue piercing.

THERAPIST: What were you expecting me to say?

PATIENT: That it makes me look crazy.

THERAPIST: What do you want people to think?

PATIENT: I just want people to accept me the way I am.

THERAPIST: Right ... that's why I didn't say anything, because I didn't want you to think that all I saw was the tongue piercing. It's you I am trying to get to know.

PATIENT: So you aren't going to tell me what you think?

THERAPIST: Well, if you push me, my first thought was "That must have really hurt when you put it in!"

Here the therapist is balancing being nonjudgmental with being genuine.

It is vital for the therapist to project self-confidence about his or her ability to help the adolescent. We have learned from experience that many adolescents easily recognize when a therapist is overwhelmed by the severity of their problems—particularly their suicidality. If the adolescent senses apprehension or discomfort on the part of the therapist, this may serve to increase the teen's belief that he or she is beyond help. In turn, this may also lead the teen to be less disclosing with the therapist, out of a belief that the therapist "couldn't handle it anyway." This does not imply that it is the sole responsibility of the therapist to solve all of the teen's problems. Rather, it is of the utmost importance for the therapist to communicate to the teen that he or she is committed to working together toward resolving the teen's problems.

Self-confidence also includes feeling secure enough to share with a patient or family when the therapist is not sure about the next move. The therapist should convey confidence that together they will be able to figure out what the next step should be.

CASE EXAMPLE

George was a 16-year-old boy who had been in treatment for depression and suicidal thoughts and behavior for over a year. Approximately 2 months ago, his depression worsened. He had a 4-day inpatient hospitalization followed by 3 weeks at the partial hospital program, during which time he actively participated in treatment and his mood improved. He returned to his outpatient therapist and was preparing to go on a 2-week school trip to a foreign country. His parents and the school wanted to know if it was safe for him to go on the trip. The therapist suggested that they think it through together. The therapist helped the teen and parents to evaluate the benefits and risks of going and of not going. The therapist was direct with the family that this was not an easy decision, and that there was no obvious and completely right answer. In this way, the therapist helped guide the family and teen to a decision that was consistent with the patient's needs and therapeutic goals. This example illustrates the importance of the therapist conveying confidence in his- or herself, and also in the therapeutic process.

The ability to be straightforward, direct, and assertive with the adolescent allows for productive communication in therapy. For example, if the patient shares information in passing that is concerning to the therapist, and then immediately wants to move on to discuss another topic in session, it is the therapist's responsibility to communicate concern to the patient—by saying, for example, "This seems like an important issue. I think we should make sure to focus on this today. Any reason why we shouldn't?" When the therapist is direct with the adolescent, it increases the likelihood that the adolescent will in turn be direct with the therapist. Furthermore, many depressed and suicidal teens lack skills in appropriate assertiveness. The therapist's in-session behavior serves as a model for the teen to learn a more direct communication style.

Flexibility is also important for dealing with patients whose clinical state can change frequently. Flexibility allows the therapist to be attuned to the teen's fluctuating needs and priorities, and to respond accordingly. The ability to be flexible allows the therapist to validate the adolescent's *current* concerns, rather than forging ahead with a pre-set agenda. Together, the therapist and teen can decide on a direction. Since many suicidal and depressed patients engage in "all or nothing" thinking, modeling flexibility is helpful as well.

Finally, the appropriate "use of self" is a potent strategy in working with teens. The use of self can involve the therapist's incorporation of his or her own personal assets in treatment. For example, a strong sense of humor, skill in using metaphors, and personal knowledge about a topic of particular importance to the teen (e.g., music, movies, skiing) can all be effectively incorporated into treatment. We do not mean to imply that there is a certain personality style that is optimal for the treatment of depressed and suicidal teens. Rather, we mean that the therapist should be comfortable with him- or herself. A therapist who is uncomfortable with major aspects of his or her personality will have difficulty being genuine and staying calm in the face of crises. Often, our professional training discourages us from bringing our authentic personal style into the therapeutic relationship. We may be taught that in order to be effective therapists, we need to create a professional persona that does not allow or make room for our own true personality. In our experience, adolescents respond best to therapists who bring genuineness to the relationship. Teens know when we are not being ourselves. They respond in kind. They will not disclose or fully engage in the therapeutic process if they feel the therapist is not being real. The collaborative nature of this treatment lends itself well to incorporating a real partnership between the teen and the therapist. All of the role plays we offer are reflections of our own styles. It is important for individual therapists to incorporate this information into their *own* genuine style, rather than just trying to imitate the examples in this book.

Although we believe that all of these interpersonal skills can be learned and developed, it is also true that working with depressed, suicidal adolescents is not for every therapist. It is important for each therapist to discern when he or she needs to further develop these interpersonal skills and when working with this population may simply be a poor fit. Part of being a good therapist is the ability to recognize one's own therapeutic strengths and weaknesses. In so doing, the therapist can determine which populations best fit with his or her style. After all, no therapist is best suited to treat every type of patient.

THE THERAPEUTIC RELATIONSHIP

The therapeutic relationship develops optimally when the therapist combines technical with interpersonal skills in the collaborative treatment with the adolescent. In order for a solid therapeutic relationship to be established, the patient must feel safe, validated, and able to trust that the therapist has his or her best interests in mind. Most psychotherapy research indicates that the therapeutic relationship is one of the most potent predictors of treatment outcome. The building blocks of a good therapeutic relationship include the interpersonal skills described above. In addition, there need to be clear rules about confidentiality, the role of parents in the treatment, and the expectations of both the therapist and the patient. There also needs to be a way for the therapist and patient to address what is happening if things are not going well, so that the relationship can be repaired or enhanced. As such, it is clear that the therapeutic relationship serves as the foundation for the entire treatment. We cannot underscore enough the importance of attending to the relationship between therapist and teen. We describe techniques for building and enhancing the therapeutic relationship in Chapter 4.

There will be times when we as therapists make mistakes. For example, unexpected circumstances arise that can cause even the most organized and timely therapist to be late for a scheduled session. When these things occur, we encourage therapists to be straightforward with the teen. This is a good opportunity to model for patients and their families how to appropriately take responsibility when mistakes happen, and to respectfully apologize and acknowledge the impact their behavior has on the patient and family.

To summarize, we have described three important components for the successful treatment of depressed and suicidal adolescents: (1) the organizational environment, (2) the individual as therapist, and (3) the development of a positive therapeutic relationship between the therapist and the teen. Attention to each element is important in order to maximize the treatment outcome. In the chapters that follow, we describe these necessary skills, and how to use them to build and maintain a therapeutic relationship.

KEY POINTS

- The treatment team provides:
  - Multidisciplinary approach
  - Supportive environment
  - Consultation regarding risk management
- Primary functions of supervision:
  - Enhancing therapist's skills set
  - Optimizing use of therapist's own characteristics
  - Providing support and encouragement
- Recommendations for 24-hour backup:
  - Utilize organizational ("in-house") resources
  - Utilize community resources
- Essential therapist characteristics:
  - Collaborative in nature
  - Genuine and nonjudgmental
  - Flexible
  - Confident and assertive
- The therapeutic partnership serves as the foundation for treatment

CHAPTER 4

Getting Started

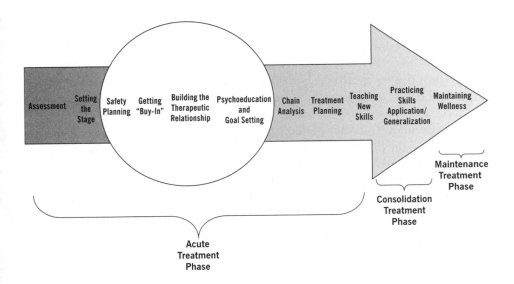

WHAT YOU WILL LEARN IN THIS CHAPTER

- How to structure a session.
- How to create a safety plan.
- Determining appropriate level of care.
- Guidelines for discussing confidentiality.
- Getting the teen's buy-in to treatment.
- Building the therapeutic relationship.
- Patient and family psychoeducation.
- Goal setting.

Now that the therapist has conducted a thorough assessment and has otherwise set the stage for treatment, the acute phase of treatment with a depressed and suicidal adolescent can begin in earnest. This chapter focuses specifically on structuring a session, negotiating the safety plan, determining the appropriate level of care, discussing confidentiality, getting the teen's buy-in for treatment, building the therapeutic relationship, and conducting psychoeducation with the teen and family.

HOW TO STRUCTURE A SESSION

Agenda Setting

Since the foundation of CBT is collaborative empiricism, it is important to ask the teen for feedback and ideas about each aspect of therapy. Setting the agenda together for each session is an important way to establish the collaborative partnership. The therapist and teen should mutually set priorities for each session, which will help engage the teen in treatment. Initially the teen may not be sure of what to put on the agenda, and the therapist should be prepared to model and socialize the teen to what type of items are appropriate for the agenda. Further into treatment, the agenda will include a summary of the teen's experiences since the last session. This should include a summary and brief review of last session, review of homework, check-in regarding current mood, suicidality check, and safety plan review.

Here are some suggestions regarding how to set the agenda:

- "Is there anything on your mind you'd like to focus on today?"
- "Do you have some ideas of what you would like to put on the agenda for our session today?"
- "Did you have some experiences over the past week that you would like to discuss?"

The agenda may also include the discussion of successes that may have occurred during the week, or administrative issues (e.g., scheduling, insurance). We have found it best to set the agenda first and then to collaboratively decide on priorities that are suitable for the available time.

Summarizing a Session and Getting Feedback

At the beginning of each session, we find it helpful to ask the teen to summarize his or her recollection of the previous session. Additionally, we recommend asking the teen for feedback on the last session, including thoughts and feelings.

Throughout the session, it is useful to summarize what has been discussed so far. When a teen is very depressed, his or her concentration may be impaired. Sometimes emotionally charged discussions may also interfere with the teen's ability to process or take in the information discussed. Therefore, after any lengthy discussion or important points, the therapist may want to ask the teen to summarize or highlight his or her understanding of what has been discussed. This also helps the therapist determine whether he or she is on the same page as the teen.

At the end of each session, the therapist can also elicit feedback about the session. The therapist can also provide his or her thoughts about how the session went. *Exchanging* feedback is an effective method for illustrating the collaborative nature of the treatment. Occasionally, the therapist and teen together can take a step back and discuss overall progress of the treatment.

NEGOTIATING THE SAFETY PLAN

Treatment of depressed and suicidal adolescents starts with safety planning. *Safety planning* refers to the prevention and management of risk factors that are likely to contribute in the longer term to suicidal risk.

In order to reach the point of teaching new skills, the therapist must first work with the patient to establish immediate safety. In our model of treatment, we achieve this by negotiating a safety plan—the construction of the safety plan involves the reduction of *imminent* suicidal risk.

What Is a Safety Plan?

A safety plan is a hierarchically arranged list of strategies that the patient agrees to employ in the event of a suicidal crisis. The development of a safety plan is considered one of the most critical parts of the assessment and treatment of suicidal youth, and involves collaboration between the therapist, patient, and family. We recommend that the therapist and teen write out the steps of the safety plan as they create the plan together (see Figure 4.1). The safety plan is one of the first interventions a therapist employs with a suicidal teen. Safety plans serve to increase the patient's sense of control by demonstrating that he or she can get through suicidal thoughts and urges without acting on them.

FIGURE 4.1. Sample safety plan format.

Professionals who I can ask for help:

My therapist: _____ Phone #: _____

Hospital ER: _____ Phone #: _____

Crisis hotline/Other: _____

Arrows (left to right):

Setting the Stage: Making the environment safe

Recognizing Warning Signs

Internal Strategies: Things I can do on my own

External Strategies: People who can help distract me

External Strategies: Adults I can ask for help

How Does a Therapist Negotiate a Safety Plan?

A safety plan is tailor-made for each adolescent based on his or her unique circumstances. Negotiating a safety plan can help determine the appropriate level of care: the inability to collaborate on a safety plan indicates that a higher level than outpatient care is needed. However, care should be taken to avoid the use of coercion when negotiating the safety plan with the adolescent so as not to mask the adolescent's suicidal risk.

To illustrate, Kathy, age 15, had a history of two prior suicide attempts that led to psychiatric hospitalizations. On three additional occasions, after disclosing suicidal ideation with a plan to her previous treatment provider, she was immediately hospitalized. Kathy reported that she hated going to the hospital and would do anything to avoid it. Kathy presented for a therapy session this morning, at which time she reported worsening depressive symptoms. We will use Kathy's case to illustrate first a coercive approach, and then a collaborative approach, to exploring current suicide risk.

Coercive Approach

THERAPIST: It really stinks that you are feeling worse this week. I am wondering if you have experienced any return of suicidal thoughts?

KATHY: Why, are you going to send me to the hospital?

THERAPIST: That depends on what you say.

KATHY: Well, then, no!

THERAPIST: Well, when I hear that type of "no," I must assume it really means you *are* suicidal but you are thinking I might send you to the hospital if you say yes ... and I know you hate the hospital.

KATHY: No, that's not it at all!

THERAPIST: Then you need to convince me that you are safe before you can go home.

KATHY: OK. I am fine. I have my safety plan right here and I know who I would call if I need anything.

THERAPIST: OK, so we are good?

KATHY: Yep.

Collaborative Approach

THERAPIST: It really stinks that you are feeling worse this week. I am wondering if you have experienced any return of suicidal thoughts?

KATHY: Why, are you going to send me to the hospital?

THERAPIST: I know you don't like the hospital and that you and I have an agreement to work hard together to keep you out of the hospital. Do you feel differently about our plan today?

KATHY: No, not really. I am just worried if I tell you what I am thinking, then you will make my mom take me to the ER.

THERAPIST: Oh, I see. So you were thinking somehow I would be the one to make the decision. Actually Kathy, I would prefer you and I make that decision together.

KATHY: Oh, so you don't think I need to go to the hospital?

THERAPIST: Well, let's figure it out together. How would we know if you needed to go?

What Are the Strategies Involved in Creating a Safety Plan?

The first strategy involved in developing a safety plan is to eliminate the availability of lethal means in the patient's environment. This may include firearms, ammunition, pills, and sharp objects (e.g., knives). Next, a no-harm agreement is negotiated between the adolescent, parents, and therapist that, in the event the adolescent has suicidal urges, he or she will defer acting on suicidal thoughts and urges for a specified period of time. During this period, the adolescent agrees to try other potential solutions. The therapist then works with the patient to develop a plan for coping with suicidal thoughts and urges. The patient is asked to identify the warning signs of a suicidal crisis. Warning signs may include specific thoughts (e.g., "I hate my life"), emotions (e.g., despair), and/or behaviors (e.g., social isolation).

Vulnerability factors that decrease the threshold for suicidality for that adolescent may also be identified. Examples of vulnerability factors include certain social situations, events, life themes, substance use, or sleep difficulties. The therapist may negotiate with the teen to avoid (if possible) activities and/or situations that increase suicidality.

The safety plan involves a stepwise increase in level of intervention from internal coping strategies to external strategies. Primarily, patients are encouraged to consider internal strategies—that is, coping skills they can employ without the assistance of other people. As a therapeutic strategy, it is important right from the beginning of treatment to have teens try to cope on their own with their suicidal thoughts, even if it is just for a brief time. The therapist can ask, "What can you do, on your own, if you get suicidal again to help yourself not act on urges?" Typical examples of internal coping strategies for adolescents involve distractions like listening to music, going for a jog, watching television (e.g., cartoons, comedy), or taking a shower. In the safety plan, the therapist should help the patient identify a few of these strategies that he or she would agree to use in order of priority (starting with what is easiest and/or most likely to be effective). As patients learn new skills during treatment, additional coping strategies should be included in the safety plan. Although the safety plan is developed at the beginning of treatment, it is reviewed and modified in subsequent sessions, as an increasingly larger number of coping skills become available to patients throughout treatment. Next, the therapist and patient can explore and problem-solve potential barriers to utilizing internal coping strategies. For example, the therapist might ask, "What might get in the way of you thinking of these activities or doing them if you think of them? How can we remove those obstacles?"

The therapist should inform the teen that if one step in the safety plan is unavailable, he or she should not stop and wait until it becomes available. Similarly, if a strategy proves unhelpful, that does not give the teen permission to give up. Instead, in the event that internal strategies do not work to avert the suicidal crisis, patients should next identify in the safety plan key contact people who can be enlisted to help. Ideally, contact people include at least one of the teen's parents. In the event the teen is not willing to include a parent as a contact person, the therapist should collaborate with the teen and parents to identify alternative responsible adults. Together, a plan should be made for sharing this information with the contact person, and details of the plan should be conveyed to him or her. In the event that one contact person cannot be reached, we encourage the teen to develop a list with multiple people. Commonly, teens will first identify a peer as their primary contact person. It is important to allow the teen to include whomever he or she identifies as a trusted contact person, with the understanding that being a contact person is a big responsibility that could be overwhelming to a teen. Therefore, the safety plan must also include a responsible level-headed adult.

The names and phone numbers of the contact people are identified. This list includes contact information for the therapist and other mental health professionals involved in the adolescent's treatment. The name, address, and phone number of the nearest psychiatric emergency room should also be included. Sometimes teens are reluctant to contact a professional for fear that the professional will immediately suggest hospitalization or, alternatively, will not be available to speak with them. In some instances, a role play could be used in which the patient practices calling the therapist, and the therapist responds to the patient's concerns. Following the role play, the therapist asks the patient for feedback to assess how well the role play addressed the patient's concerns.

The contact people on the safety plan can be utilized by the patient in a number of ways. Patients can initially reach out to peers for distraction. However, if this is not sufficient to manage the patient's suicidal urges, then the teen should enlist the help of responsible adults in the safety plan. This may range from disclosing how badly the teen feels to disclosing suicidality. There can be a stepwise progression from including those in the natural support group (e.g., parents) to professionals.

Troubleshooting

The therapist and patient should review each step of the plan and collaboratively problem-solve any potential roadblocks to implementation. The therapist may ask questions to determine patients' expectations about the effectiveness of each step. For example, the therapist may ask: "On a scale of 1 (not at all likely) to 10 (very likely), how likely do you think you would be to do this step during a time of crisis?" If the patient indicates that he or she is not at all likely, or unsure if he or she would be able to engage in an activity on the safety plan, then there are several strategies that can be employed: (1) check to see if the patient understands the rationale for a particular step and provide clarification if necessary; (2) discuss possible roadblocks that may prevent a specific skill from being used, and then use problem-solving skills to address them; and (3) collaboratively generate an alternative strategy that could be used that the patient can agree to do (expand the safety plan).

This safety plan may be reworked or revised in any way that the therapist and patient see fit. The therapist and patient should also discuss where the patient will keep the written safety plan and how it will be retrieved during a period of crisis. One way of ensuring that patients have this information on hand is to give them small coping cards that they can carry with them. These cards may consist of very short phrases to remind the patient of the specific steps that are described in the safety plan (see Figure 4.2).

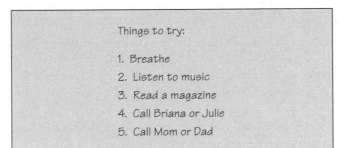

Things to try:

1. Breathe
2. Listen to music
3. Read a magazine
4. Call Briana or Julie
5. Call Mom or Dad

FIGURE 4.2. Sample coping card.

Ongoing Development of the Safety Plan

It is important to link the safety plan to the patient's suicidal behavior and precursors of suicidal behavior. The patient should understand that the plan is fluid, and that skills and strategies will be added to the plan as the patient learns more throughout treatment. In the beginning of treatment, the safety plan may simply consist of an agreement to call emergency contacts and/or very basic coping strategies. The therapist can review on an ongoing basis what has and has not worked for the adolescent, and modify based on these experiences.

The Family's Role in the Safety Plan

Ideally, the safety plan is first developed with the patient individually. Then the therapist and patient can collaborate on how the family can be helpful in supporting the patient in implementing the safety plan. It may be helpful to discuss with the teen what he or she would and would not like to have shared with the family. Together with the patient, agree on how to present the safety plan to the family.

Family cooperation in the development of a safety plan is extremely important. First, family members are often resources in the safety plan. Second, adults need to secure the environment to make it as safe as possible for the suicidal youth. One study highlights specific elements of psychoeducation regarding access to firearms that may be critical in decreasing risk—namely, talking directly to the gun owner, understanding why the gun owner has the gun in the house, and negotiating ways to make the gun more secure rather than insisting on removal of the gun (even though the latter is ideal).

Finally, another important family component to the safety plan is the negotiation of a truce around "hot topics," or other possible precipitants to future suicidality. This truce gives permission for the patient and parents to table issues that trigger conflict until they have learned how to disagree without having it lead to suicidal behavior. Once the family agrees to the truce, it is additionally important to rehearse with the family what each member will do if the truce breaks down (e.g., agree or give permission to leave the room so as not to continue the argument). In subsequent sessions, the therapist should check in with the family regarding the status of the truce.

CASE EXAMPLE

THERAPIST: So the issue of you dating Joe seems to be a big source of conflict for you and your family. From us talking today, we have identified that this conflict frequently leads to suicidal thoughts for you. Therefore, I was hoping we could arrive at an agreement about how to handle this topic. I am not saying we don't need to solve this problem. However, at least until we have you engaged in treatment and your mood is less depressed, could we agree on temporarily tabling discussion of this topic between you and your parents? What I mean by this is choosing to put it on the back burner and agreeing to a temporary truce. What do you think?

TAMEKA: OK, but what does that mean exactly?

PARENTS: Yes, a truce makes sense, but how do we do that?

THERAPIST: Good, so let us move on to discuss what a truce would look like. Mom and Dad, what kind of temporary compromise would you suggest?

PARENTS: Well, we would rather Tameka not see Joe at all, but we realize he is important to her, so how about if she can talk with him on the phone after school for an hour each day and see him at our house but only on weekends.

THERAPIST: Tameka, how does that sound to you?

TAMEKA: I am OK with that, at least for now.

THERAPIST: Great. It is clear to me that you and your parents are really invested in working this out together. I know this is a tough issue, so maybe we should think together on what might get in the way of keeping the "truce" and how you could respond it if breaks down.

TAMEKA: If they are mad at me about something else, then they will not let him come over.

THERAPIST: Yes, I agree that would make it difficult to keep the truce. Mom and Dad, what do you think?

PARENTS: Yes, it will be hard, but we can try our best to stick to this agreement. However, we expect you to keep your end of the deal too. That means no sneaking out to see him and respecting the time limit on phone calls with him.

TAMEKA: I can do that.

DETERMINING APPROPRIATE LEVEL OF CARE

One of the therapist's primary tasks is to determine whether the adolescent can safely be managed as an outpatient. A patient with active suicidal ideation with a clear method who cannot agree to a safety plan should be managed in a more intensive setting. Patients who are acutely psychotic, manic, in a mixed state, or substance-dependent also are best managed in a more intensive setting. Patients who are currently being abused, or at significant and ongoing risk for abuse, should be removed from the home, although not necessarily hospitalized. If the patient and family refuse admission to a higher level of care, the therapist needs to weigh the needs of the patient versus the possible damage to the relationship that would occur if the therapist chose to hospitalize a patient against the family's will. This course of action should be taken only if the therapist feels that the patient's (or another's) life is in immediate danger.

With the current state of mental health care, inpatient hospitalizations are frequently short term and focused on ensuring basic safety of the patient. Despite the limitations of inpatient treatment, hospitalization continues to be the recommended standard of care for patients experiencing acute psychosis, mania, and/or acute suicidality with imminent risk to harm self or others. Suicidal adolescents have been shown to be at particularly high risk for suicidal behavior during the period immediately following discharge from a psychiatric hospital. Often, adolescents experience a reprieve from psychosocial stress while in the hospital, thus making the transition out of the hospital and back to daily life a difficult period. Therefore, upon discharge from the hospital, we recommend consideration of an intermediate level of care (see below) prior to returning to or starting traditional weekly outpatient treatment.

In many areas of the country, teens have access to intermediate levels of care such as intensive outpatient (IOP) and partial hospitalization programs, which require more intensive care than weekly outpatient treatment, but less intensive care than hospitalization. These types of programs should also be considered for patients who are not responding to traditional outpatient treatment and continue to exhibit suicidality and/or significant functional impairment (e.g., are not attending school regularly).

Additionally, adjunctive psychosocial services may be available to support the teens and their families. We often collaborate with services such as case management and family-based treatment.

BUILDING RAPPORT DURING THE FIRST SESSION

Many teens make up their minds early about the treatment—whether they like the therapist, and whether they are even coming back or not for another session. Therefore, it is essential to *hook* the teen during this first session.

Often, teens come to the first session feeling like they are "on the hot seat," or as if they are "under a microscope." By taking the lead and orienting the teen to what will happen in the session, the therapist allows the teen to settle in and feel less scrutinized. The first part of a first therapy session may sound something like this:

> THERAPIST: Hello, Ginny, my name is Kim. It's nice to meet you. Is it OK if I spend a few minutes telling you a little bit about what I thought we might do today?
>
> GINNY: Yeah, sure, I don't care ...
>
> THERAPIST: I was hoping we could start by getting to know each other a bit. I am also really interested in hearing your take on what brings you here and what your thoughts are on what could be helpful.

Now, we recommend that the therapist spend some time talking about the patient's life. In order to get to know her, the therapist may ask about things like where she goes to school, what kind of music she likes, activities and interests, friends, and anything else in her life that is important to her. This helps her know that the therapist is interested in her as an individual, not just her problems.

One of the first discussions the therapist has when working with a new patient involves the patient's feelings about beginning treatment. It is important for the therapist to understand how he or she came to be referred at this time. We often hear teens report that someone else "made them come to treatment." The therapist should communicate a respect for the teen's level of apprehension, and encourage him or her to ask questions and express any concerns. This stance by the therapist acknowledges the teen's important developmental need for increasing autonomy and control.

CONFIDENTIALITY

In order for teens to work effectively in therapy, it is imperative that a trusting relationship be established with the therapist. Many teens may not have had the experience of a trusting relationship with an adult before and therefore have the expectation that all adult relationships will be of an authoritarian nature. Even if the teen does not have this expectation, he or she certainly will not usually come to therapy expecting a collaborative partnership. We have found this to be a critical element for building the therapeutic relationship. In order for trust to be established, the groundwork of confidentiality must be firmly established.

Therefore, the therapist initiates a discussion about the ground rules regarding confidentiality in the first session. This helps the teen feel a sense of trust and privacy. However, we do not promise an unrealistic or unhelpful amount of confidentiality. The following are some useful guidelines. First, we begin by asking the teen what he or she knows or understands about confidentiality. We then go on to explain that the majority of things we will talk about in therapy will remain between us (i.e., the therapist and other members of the team) and the teen. The therapist could begin as follows: "If you tell me something about a strong feeling you have about a friend or family member, such as 'I hate my mom and I will never talk with her again,' then that is clearly something that would stay just between you and me." However, we do not promise absolute confidentiality to the teen. Rather, we aim to help the teen understand that life-threatening issues that may necessitate a change in the treatment plan must be shared with his or her parents. For example: "If you tell me you are going to kill yourself, or that you are being abused, I cannot keep that private. However, before we talk with your parents, we will need to discuss *how* we should tell them." The key element is that the patient and therapist will collaborate to figure out how best to present this information to the parents.

CASE EXAMPLE

THERAPIST: Alex, I really appreciate your honesty about your current suicidal thoughts of overdosing with Tylenol. I am sorry it's been such a difficult week for you. I am also worried about you and I am thinking that we need some extra supports right now. Is your mom aware how badly you are feeling now?

ALEX: No. She is so busy at work right now, I barely even saw her this week. She can't help.

THERAPIST: I know your mom is really busy—but I also know she really wants to know from us what's going on and how she can be helpful. What are your thoughts about this?

ALEX: It would be good if she could help, but I am afraid she will get mad at me ...

THERAPIST: Yes, that could happen, but I am wondering if we could try to talk with her together, if that could make a difference. Maybe you and I could figure out the best way to approach your mom and then practice together how we would express our current concerns around safety. Then, we will bring her back and talk with her together. How's that sound?

ALEX: OK.

What If the Teen Says "No"

If the teen is unwilling to talk with a parent about current safety concerns, it is important for the therapist to express concern directly and honestly to the patient. The therapist should be willing to hear all about the teen's reasons for not wanting to divulge the current suicidality to the parent, and validate these concerns. Most of the time, the teen's reasons are quite valid. At the same time, the therapist needs to remain consistent and "stay the course" around the agreement made regarding the limits of confidentiality. At this time, it can be helpful for the therapist to remind the teen of the agreement.

CASE EXAMPLE

THERAPIST: I am in this with you. I am on your team. However, I can't help you if you aren't alive. So, our first priority always will be to keep you alive. So, *how* are we going to let your mom know about our current concerns? [Notice that the therapist is not focusing on *if* the information will be shared, but instead on *how* the information will be shared.]

LEAH: I don't want her to know—she will freak out like always and not let me go to the dance Saturday night.

THERAPIST: So, you are worried about her reaction. I see why that would be a concern. Is there a way that you and I together could let her know about last night's increase in suicidal thoughts, yet at the same time reassure her that you did not do anything to hurt yourself and continue to be committed to the safety plan? This way, we can help her see a couple things. One, you are letting us know when you have suicidal thoughts, and secondly, you are able to keep yourself safe. In many ways this could be a good opportunity to show your mom that you are really working hard in treatment and a bump in the road does not mean you are back where you started. You handled this very differently than you might have in the past. What do you think?

LEAH: Yeah, it sounds OK, but I still worry she will want to keep me home this weekend.

THERAPIST: Do you think it makes a difference *how* we present it to her?

LEAH: Probably so. Could you start off by telling her that I am better than I used to be?

THERAPIST: Sure, I think that's a great idea to start out with the positives.

LEAH: It will go better if she hears it from you, instead of just me ...

THERAPIST: We can do that. Let's meet with her together and I will start out with emphasizing the positives, then together we can let her know about last night's bump in the road.

This process can be tedious and time-consuming, but it *cannot* be rushed. Negotiating with the teen is critical, both about the specifics of the safety plan and how the information will be shared with the family. The danger of rushing ahead without the teen's buy-in (at least a partial buy-in) is that it can permanently damage trust and set a noncollaborative tone for the remainder of treatment. Successfully and collaboratively negotiating the management of the teen's current suicidality can help to solidify the therapeutic relationship.

GETTING THE TEEN'S BUY-IN

Despite the fact that most teens do not self-refer, we encourage the therapist to help the teen identify areas to focus on in treatment that will ultimately increase his or her sense of autonomy and control; we call this *getting the teen's buy-in*. For example, the therapist might ask, "What changes would you like to see for yourself or your family?" It is critical that the teen is "on board the bus" before "pulling out of the station." This can be achieved by presenting a solid rationale for how therapy can be useful to the teen in achieving his or her self-defined goals, and then soliciting the teen's feedback.

CASE EXAMPLE

THERAPIST: So, Ginny, whose idea was it for you to come see me today?

GINNY: Certainly not mine. My mom thinks I am depressed.

THERAPIST: What do you think?

GINNY: I think my mom is overreacting. If she would just back off and give me some space, I am sure I would feel better.

THERAPIST: That sounds reasonable.

GINNY: I know I am messing up in school, but I am sure I can take care of it on my own.

THERAPIST: Now that you are here, how do you feel about talking with me?

GINNY: It's OK. I don't think I need a shrink or anything, but it's fine.

THERAPIST: So, the points you have raised, Ginny, are very good ones. Sometimes parents do get worried when they see any change in how their teens act. This can be irritating for the teen. However, sometimes changes do reflect a potential problem. So, I am wondering if you and I could get to know each other a bit and try and sort out together what's really going on. Later, you and I could share some of our conclusions with your mom. How's that sound?

It is also important for the therapist to inquire into the teen's beliefs about, and previous experiences with, mental health treatment. By doing so, the therapist begins to gather valuable information about the teen's perceptions of self and the prospect of change. For example, teens often come to therapy with the notion that being referred for mental health treatment means they are "messed up" and destined to have a dysfunctional life.

Some additional questions you may want to ask include:

- "Have you been in treatment before? If so, what was it like?"
- "What did you like/dislike about the previous experience?"
- "What things worked/didn't work?"
- "If you haven't been in therapy before, what are your thoughts about therapy?"

- "Do you know anyone who is or has ever been in therapy?"
- "What do you think it means about someone if they go to therapy?"

BUILDING THE THERAPEUTIC RELATIONSHIP

Recall from Chapter 3 that the therapeutic relationship requires the therapist to utilize not only technical skills but also interpersonal skills—particularly the ability to collaborate, defer judgment, and project self-confidence, as well as assertiveness, flexibility, and appropriate use of self. The manner in which each of these interpersonal skills may be utilized to build the relationship with the teen is detailed in this section.

Building a solid therapeutic relationship with the teen entails collaboration on the parts of both therapist and teen. The therapist should communicate to the teen the importance of working together as a team toward his or her goals ("*We* will work together on goals and strategies as well as decisions about how and when to involve your family.") The use of the word *we* communicates and establishes an alliance between the therapist and the teen, without promising absolute confidentiality (see the section above on confidentiality). Ultimately, the therapist aims to communicate to the teen that the therapist and teen are on the same page, that this is the teen's treatment, and that he or she is in charge.

The ability to defer judgment often comes into play while hearing the teen's thoughts about being in treatment. It is important for the therapist to validate the adolescent's perspective, even if the therapist does not agree. Some therapists may experience a desire to move quickly toward change by offering the teen suggestions, ideas, or reassurance. Others may find a strong desire to prioritize their own treatment agenda over whatever it is that the teen is bringing. This experience is especially common for therapists dealing with suicidal teens. Clearly, many therapists feel pressured to push for change when the issue of safety is so prominent. Yet, before the issue of change can be effectively addressed, the teen needs to know the therapist has heard and accepted him or her.

Acceptance is best fostered by utilizing one's skills in deferring judgment to establish and maintain a nonjudgmental environment. For therapy to be most effective, the teen needs to experience therapy as a place he or she can come and be able to express any thoughts, feelings, and experiences without risk of negative consequences (e.g., punishment, shame, invalidation). Many teens are accustomed to experiencing other adults in their lives, even well-intentioned adults, as judgmental. When therapists notice their own strong judgments about or disapproval of the teen's experience in treatment, this indicates that the therapist needs to gather more information to better understand the teen's experience without negative judgments. Discussing the case with a supervisor or colleague may be helpful for gaining perspective and increasing the therapist's ability to maintain a nonjudgmental stance. Taking the time to listen without judgment does not equal agreement with or approval of what the teen is sharing. Rather, it demonstrates acceptance of the teen and positions the therapist to facilitate future change. This is often an initial stumbling block for therapists. When a teen presents with a distressing problematic behavior (e.g., superficial self-cutting with a razor blade), it can be difficult for the therapist to resist the urge to rush in with an intervention geared toward immediate extinction of the problematic behavior. Clearly, these types of problems are difficult for the therapist to hear without taking action. However, for meaningful change to occur, the teen first must feel that the therapist understands and does not judge him or her negatively for the behavior. Let's take the example of Jenna, age 15, who was superficially cutting her arms with a razor blade. First, we will highlight a more judgmental exchange with the therapist, followed by a nonjudgmental interaction.

Judgmental

THERAPIST: It sounds like you really had a hard time Friday night.

JENNA: Yeah, the fight with Joe really upset me and I couldn't stand it. The only thing I could think of to help me feel better was to cut myself.

THERAPIST: Seriously, how could that make you feel better?

JENNA: I don't know ... it just does. I did feel better.

THERAPIST: But now you are going to have another scar. You couldn't think of one other thing to do instead?

Nonjudgmental

THERAPIST: It sounds like you really had a hard time Friday night.

JENNA: Yeah, the fight with Joe really upset me and I couldn't stand it. The only thing I could think of to help me feel better was to cut myself.

THERAPIST: Yeah, when you are that upset, it can be really hard to think of anything else.

JENNA: Yeah, that is exactly what happened. Afterwards, I did remember other things I could have tried that might have helped.

THERAPIST: Right, your brain went straight to cutting because we know that for at least the short run, it does help you feel better. Unfortunately, you and I have learned that cutting does not help in the long run because you end up feeling bad about the choice and you don't like the scars.

Perhaps more important than the content of the first session is the style in which the content is delivered. Over the years, we have found it to be especially important for therapists working with this population to develop a style that allows them to share basic information about themselves while also maintaining professional boundaries. This helps humanize the therapist in the teen's eyes by demonstrating that the therapist is a real person whose daily life includes positive and negative experiences like everyone else's. Many times teens say, "You wouldn't know. Your life is perfect." Sharing glimpses of one's own challenges enables the teen to connect with the therapist on a genuine level. This does *not* mean that the therapist should disclose personal or private information about his or her life (e.g., history of abuse, treatment, substance use). Instead, the therapist can use benign personal examples to model effective or skillful management of life's problems. Remember, the therapist is in an influential position to model for the teen how to solve real-life problems. The following example illustrates this principle:

THERAPIST: I know what you mean—it is difficult to solve problems when you are really upset. The other day, I was late for work and had a very important meeting with my boss and wouldn't you know, I went to my car only to find a "boot" on the tire. [*Teen laughs.*] How embarrassing. I was so mad and frustrated. I wanted to go back to bed and pull the covers over my head.

TEEN: So, what did you do?

THERAPIST: I stood there for a minute, shaking my head and telling myself I should have paid the parking meter tickets on time. But then I realized I couldn't go back and change that now. So, I took a few deep breaths and started to think about my options. First, I realized I should call my office to let my boss know I would be late. Then, I tried to figure out how I would get to work. I thought it would take too much time to get the boot removed, so I needed to figure out another way to get to work. I called my friend, who agreed to give me a ride. Once I returned home that evening, I called the number on the boot and made arrangements to pay my outstanding parking tickets and get the boot removed.

Being Present

For many therapists, our schedules and many competing responsibilities make it a challenge to focus wholly on one thing at one time. For example, therapists may have a number of families to call, or they may find themselves still thinking about the last patient, or all of the other things they have yet to finish that day, all while the next patient is sitting in front of them. Patients may notice our distraction. This is especially true with depressed adolescents, who may experience our distraction as invalidating. Thus, we underscore the importance of being present with the teen. Being present involves *really* listening and attending fully to the content and process that is occurring in the moment! There are many ways for therapists to demonstrate this—verbally, and through eye contact and body language (e.g., leaning forward, maintaining an open body stance).

As therapists, we try to take notice of times when we find ourselves thinking about other things. First, we notice our distraction and try to refocus. Sometimes, shifting body position or posture helps. If we continue to notice difficulty focusing in the moment, we may briefly highlight the temporary distraction (e.g., "Oh, Mike, I apologize, my mind just wandered somewhere else—I was thinking about something else I have to do later today. I really want to hear what happened yesterday— could you repeat that so I can really get it?"). Because teens are so good at social referencing, occasionally they will catch the therapist—before the therapist catches him- or herself—and comment on the inattention.

CASE EXAMPLE

MIKE: You sure seem out of it today. Are you even listening to me?

THERAPIST: Oh, Mike, you are completely right—I am not myself today. I don't really feel so good today—must be something going around. I might be coming down with the flu. I am sorry if it's getting in our way.

MIKE: Maybe you should go home ...

THERAPIST: Thanks, but let me see if I can try and refocus with you. Would that be OK with you?

MIKE: Sure, that is OK.

Alternatively, if the therapist knows going into the session that he or she may not be "100%," then we encourage therapists to let patients and families know this. For example:

"Hello, it's good to see you. I want to let you know that I just dealt with a pretty serious clinical emergency, and so I may not quite seem myself. I would like for us to proceed with meeting, but please excuse me if I appear a bit distracted."

Dealing with Reluctance

A special challenge in getting the teen's buy-in for treatment occurs when the teen is ambivalent or reluctant to consider the possibility of change. Such teens are often referred to as "resistant" due to their angry, irritable presentation. However, we caution therapists to avoid a power struggle, as the adolescent has valid reasons for his or her reluctance. *People do things for good reasons!* It is the therapist's role to figure out, validate, and understand (with the teen's help) the adolescent's reluctance, and subsequently address these concerns collaboratively. It is only after the reluctance has been fully validated that the therapist can move on to building a plan for change.

The therapist should first find out what the teen wants ("Is there something that you and I could work on together or that you would like to see change?"). The therapist may be able to get a "foot in the door" by finding *something* the teen wants to be different in his or her life. For example, a reluctant teen who feels forced into treatment by his mother may initially agree to work with the therapist to identify strategies for "getting Mom off his back." Some teens' apparent reluctance may be a reflection of simply not understanding how to talk in therapy, or what to even talk about. Subsequently, the therapist can present the teen with a choice of possible goals to work on together in order to help the teen begin to understand the therapeutic process, as well as to feel a sense of control.

An additional barrier to treatment engagement is hopelessness about change. Some teens do not believe that change is possible for them. They may connect and develop a relationship with the therapist, and yet steadfastly maintain the belief that no matter what they do or what the therapist tries to help them with, their lives will remain absolutely the same. The teen may say something like "I like talking with you—you are a pretty cool person, and maybe therapy helps some other people—but it's not going to work for me. My family is so messed up. This is the way it has always been, and there is no therapy in the world that can fix it." This type of response is often a reflection of adolescent patients' *external* locus of control—they believe that external factors are responsible for their current problems, and no matter what *they* do differently, they are powerless to change these external forces. Not only is it permissible to agree with such a teen's perspective, we recommend it. The therapist should avoid falling into the trap of believing that he or she must convince the teen otherwise. Therapists can validate the fact that life can be unfair; they can also acknowledge powerful external forces affecting a teen's life that he or she may be unable to change. For example, Jill, a depressed, suicidal 17-year-old teen raised by parents with drug addictions and severe psychiatric illnesses, presented as follows:

THERAPIST: It sounds like you have really been through a lot. I am really glad you are here today.

JILL: Yeah, my life has really been hard. My mother abandoned us when I was 10 and I raised my autistic sister all by myself. My dad was always out partying.

THERAPIST: So you have really had to grow up fast and carry a lot of responsibilities. I could certainly see why you would feel that life would continue to be so hard.

JILL: Right. No matter what I do, things will turn out badly for me, just like they have for my mom. She dropped out of high school when she was 17. And now I am just barely passing, so I am sure it will be the same thing for me. Even when I try, it's just too hard. There's just too much to deal with.

THERAPIST: I agree—you are up against a lot of challenges. Clearly, you have been through more in your 17 years of life than most grown-ups ever have to deal with. It is not fair. It is true that you have not had the best adult models for how you could make your life look different. On top of that, you are dealing with this depression, and you are responsible for your little sister— all while trying to be responsible for yourself. I can't imagine anybody handling this situation any better than you are.

Now that the therapist has validated the teen's experience, the stage is set to move on to identify and highlight internal factors that the teen may indeed be more likely to have power over. We illustrate by continuing the dialogue with Jill:

> THERAPIST: It is true. There are things in your life [external factors] that you do not have control over. You cannot make your mom stop using drugs or make your dad stop drinking. However, you are here now with me—and what you do have control over is you and what you do from this point on [internal factors].
>
> JILL: Yeah, but it doesn't change that I have to deal with all this crap every day.
>
> THERAPIST: You are completely right. Nothing you and I could do here will change those [external] factors in your life. I am wondering, though, if you and I could figure out some ways to begin focusing on taking care of you—and still have you feel like you are taking care of the other things that are important to you.
>
> JILL: I do seem to always take care of everyone else but myself. It would be nice to actually worry about my own self for a change. I have no idea of how I would do that, but I guess it can't hurt to try . . .

Jill's interaction with her therapist demonstrates the process of getting buy-in when the teen views her problems as stemming from external factors. However, some teens, like Malcolm, a 16-year-old, see their depression as a result of something inherently flawed within themselves—a more internally driven cause. "I have been depressed since I can remember—that's just who I am. I will always be this way." This type of response is often a reflection of an adolescent patient's *internal* locus of control.

> THERAPIST: You are right, it does seem like you have been depressed for a long time. No doubt, that would affect the way you see yourself and the future. Maybe you and I could start out by talking about clinical depression—what it is, what causes it, and, importantly, how to get better. We know you have never had treatment for this illness that you have had for a long time.
>
> MALCOLM: How do you know it's an illness and not just who I am?

THERAPIST: Good question—how about we talk together about the symptoms of depression and then you can decide for yourself?

MALCOLM: I guess.

In our experience, it is a rare teen who completely jumps on board at the very beginning of treatment and stays there. With both Jill and Malcolm, the therapist got a foot in the door by getting a partial buy-in. Typically, the teen's buy-in may fluctuate throughout treatment. Getting and keeping the teen on board is an ongoing process.

In summary, in order for teens to optimally use the therapeutic experience, they need to see how treatment could possibly work for them to change and improve their lives. In our experience, this proves to be one of the most potent predictors of a successful outcome. Without the teen's buy-in, even the best treatment, provided by the best therapist, will not succeed.

PATIENT AND FAMILY PSYCHOEDUCATION

Depression is often a chronic and recurrent disorder that requires a partnership between the therapist, patient, and family. We strongly believe education is an ongoing process, and a critical part of the partnership. Over time, the patient and family will take on more of the responsibility for the management of the disorder. The first step is to help the patient and family understand that depression is an illness and not the fault of any individual family member. The patient and family need to learn how to recognize the symptoms of depression so that they can monitor treatment response and detect recurrences in the future. They should know what an expectable course is for someone with depression and be educated about the risks and benefits of various treatment options so they can rationally select among those options. For example, if someone has already failed to respond to a medication, it is important for the clinician to explain that the selection of the next step in treatment involves some trial and error. For more specifics on conducting psychoeducation with depressed teens and their families, please see Brent and Poling (1998).

CASE EXAMPLE

A 14-year-old girl, Lynn, is brought by her parents at the request of the school because of irritability, engaging in nonsuicidal self-injurious behavior at school, decline in school performance, arguments with friends and family, and loss of interest in previously enjoyed activities. Lynn's mother says she thinks that Lynn is just a normal adolescent; she states she went through something similar during high school. Lynn's mother states that Lynn is just seeking attention and does not need treatment.

RESPONSE

Assuming that the clinician has evaluated the patient and confirmed a diagnosis of depression, the clinician can explain that there is a difference between the normal ups and downs of adolescence and depression. We can make an analogy to any other medical illness, like heart disease or diabetes. The developmental changes associated with adolescence should not result in functional impairment and self-injury. Like many other diseases, depression runs in families, and it is possible that Lynn's mother did indeed experience something similar. Most teens want and seek attention, but they do not need to resort to self-injury, constant fighting, and withdrawal from other activities.

GOAL SETTING

Once the therapist has provided initial psychoeducation to the teen and family, it is helpful to transition to a discussion of general goals for treatment. The therapist can begin by asking the teen and family for their ideas about what they most want to see change as a result of treatment. We recommend starting by asking the teen. An example of such a discussion follows:

THERAPIST: OK, so let's fast-forward about 6 months from now. How would you know treatment was helpful?

JANE: I would be feeling better.

THERAPIST: OK, sounds good. How exactly would we know you were better?

JANE: Well, I would be sleeping better and probably not be so cranky with everyone. I also wouldn't be thinking of suicide so much.

THERAPIST: I agree, those are all reasonable expectations. What else would be different in your life, like with friends, with your family, and at school?

JANE: Oh, I would be doing better in school and not having so much drama with my friends.

At this point the therapist can invite input from the parents.

> THERAPIST: Mom and Dad, what would you be hoping would be different for Jane in 6 months?
>
> MOM: I would hope she would no longer have thoughts about killing herself. That is my biggest concern. We are so worried.
>
> DAD: Me too. I just want her to be happy again. I would say things are going better when her grades come back up and she is having fun with her friends again.
>
> THERAPIST: So it sounds like you all have similar ideas about what life will look like when Jane is feeling better. How would things be different in the family?
>
> MOM: I would like to see her spending more time with us and less time alone in her room.
>
> JANE: Yeah, I could see that happening if we weren't fighting so much.
>
> DAD: Right, and more respect shown in the house.
>
> THERAPIST: So it sounds like in general, we are working toward helping Jane feel less depressed. This would mean she would be less irritable and not suicidal. Jane, you also mentioned that you want to do better in school and get along better with your friends. Finally, all of you agreed that having less family conflict would be an important outcome of treatment. Sounds good. Is there anything else we may have missed?
>
> MOM: No, I think that this covers the most important ones. Jane, do you agree?
>
> JANE: Yes, I think that is it.

To summarize, the therapist facilitates a discussion of overarching treatment goals with the teen *and* family. This allows the therapist to get input from the family, as well as to gain an understanding of their priorities in treatment.

KEY POINTS

- Structuring a session includes setting an agenda, summarizing the session, and getting feedback.
- Creation of a safety plan that involves increasing levels of intervention is a collaborative effort including the therapist, patient, and family.

- The safety plan continues to be developed throughout treatment.

- Negotiation of the safety plan informs determination of the appropriate level of care.

- To get a reluctant teen's buy-in to treatment, look for anything the teen is willing to consider working on at the outset.

- Trust in the relationship is critical; however, confidentiality in an absolute sense should not be promised to the teen.

- Due to developmental considerations, teens appreciate nonjudgmental, genuine, and open therapists.

- Psychoeducation for both the patient and family is an essential and ongoing aspect of treatment.

- Goal setting involves asking first the teen and then the parents what they most want to see change as a result of treatment.

CHAPTER 5

Chain Analysis and Treatment Planning

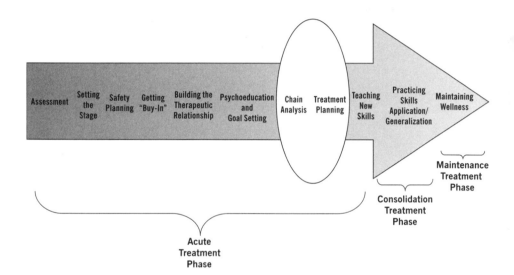

WHAT YOU WILL LEARN IN THIS CHAPTER

- What a chain analysis is.
- When to use a chain analysis.
- How to handle barriers when conducting the chain analysis.
- How to conduct a chain analysis with an adolescent.
- How to include the family in the chain analysis.
- The importance of vulnerability and protective factors.
- How to use the chain analysis to inform treatment planning.

Once the therapist, patient, and family have agreed on treatment goals, the therapist can move on to conducting the chain analysis. In this chapter we describe chain analysis, provide a rationale for it, and explain how to use the chain analysis to inform treatment planning.

WHAT IS A CHAIN ANALYSIS?

A *chain analysis* is a detailed functional analysis of *any* behavior. For our purposes, the behavior is usually a problematic behavior such as a suicide attempt, non-suicidal self-injury, alcohol or drug use, aggression, or other impulsive acts. The process of conducting the chain analysis helps the therapist and patient begin to develop an understanding of the various factors that contribute to the onset and maintenance of a specific problematic behavior. Through the identification of these factors, the therapist and patient are then positioned to identify the therapeutic interventions that will specifically target these factors.

Chain analysis has its roots in behaviorism—largely established in the early 1900s through the influential work of three theorists: Ivan Pavlov, John Watson, and B. F. Skinner. Pavlov first described classical conditioning during his work with dogs, demonstrating that an environmental stimulus (ringing a bell) could be used to stimulate a conditioned response (salivating at the sound of the bell ringing). Watson extended Pavlov's theory to apply to human behavior. Subsequently, Skinner introduced the idea of operant conditioning, whereby reinforcement leads to an increase in a desired behavior and punishment leads to a decrease in an undesired behavior.

These behavioral concepts played an influential role in informing therapeutic techniques designed to affect behavior change in a wide range of populations. For example, behavioral analysis has proven to be a particularly effective tool for helping children with developmental disabilities to acquire new skills. Similarly, behavioral analysis has long been used as a therapeutic tool for individuals with mood disordered to target difficulties in the self-regulation of affect and behavior. David Wexler (1991) described a version of chain analysis that is developmentally appropriate for adolescents. He termed this approach the *freeze frame method* for adolescents with difficulty self-regulating. In the freeze frame method, the therapist talks the teen through the incident in slow motion, as if he or she were watching a movie or TV show in slow motion. In her work at the University of Washington, Marsha Linehan (1993) utilized the chain analysis with self-injuring adults. Greg Brown and colleagues at the University of Pennsylvania (Brown et al., 2005) later used cognitive behavioral analysis with adult suicide attempters.

Often, adolescents initially cannot identify any precipitants or contributing factors to the recent problematic behavior. For example, it is not uncommon for a teen to say, "Nothing big happened the day I took the pills—I just did it—but it won't happen again." The chain analysis helps the therapist orient the teen to the idea that behaviors happen for valid reasons—even if we are not initially aware of those reasons. For example:

> "We believe that people do things for really good reasons. I am wondering if you and I could get curious together and try to figure out what those reasons may have been on that particular day?"

The process of identifying these reasons helps the therapist and teen develop a better understanding of the problem behavior. As a result, the teen can develop an increased sense of control over his or her behavior—ultimately leading the teen to believe that change is possible (see Figure 5.1).

WHEN WOULD A THERAPIST USE
A CHAIN ANALYSIS?

We encourage therapists to conduct a chain analysis in the early stage of treatment with depressed and suicidal teens. At this point in treatment the chain analysis often focuses on high-risk behaviors (e.g., self-injury, substance use, risky sex, suicidality).

In the later phase of treatment, once the risky behaviors are less frequent, we have found the chain analysis to be helpful for developing a better understanding of any particular experience (this could be a behavior or an emotion) that is distressing to the teen. For example,

---

- To help the teen identify reasons for the specific problem behavior.
- To help the teen develop increased control of the behavior.
- To enhance the teen's belief that change is possible.
- To identify vulnerabilities and skill deficits for treatment planning.

FIGURE 5.1. The reasons for conducting a chain analysis.

Julie, age 16, came to session reporting severe distress following the discovery that her best friend "hooked up with" her ex-boyfriend. Julie did not engage in self-injurious behavior (as she might have in the past), but she did experience an extremely strong and distressing emotion that she had difficulty understanding. The process of completing a chain analysis helped Julie make sense of her emotional reaction, and ultimately helped her identify ways to break links in the chain and thus to decrease her level of distress.

The chain analysis can also be used during family sessions to identify external factors associated with problem behaviors, such as family members' responses. For example, Lisa had an argument with her mother about curfew. After they had screamed and yelled at one another, Lisa stormed upstairs to her room and made superficial cuts on her arm using a razor blade. Immediately afterwards, Lisa went back downstairs and told her mother what she had done. At that point, her mother apologized. Next, Lisa apologized. The tension between them was eliminated, they hugged, and there was no further discussion of the curfew. This example shows how a problem behavior may be reinforced inadvertently by the reactions of others. Specific skills for intervening with clinical scenarios such as these will be detailed in Chapters 6 and 7.

HOW TO HANDLE OBSTACLES WHEN CONDUCTING A CHAIN ANALYSIS

In our experience, many adolescents are initially reluctant to go back and recount their story. The following are some common reasons teens give for not wanting to review the "chain of events," as well as some suggestions for how the therapist might respond:

TEEN: I would never do it again. I'll just get upset again if I talk about it.

THERAPIST: You are right. It can be very difficult to talk about such upsetting situations. I can see why you would rather not. If I were you, I probably wouldn't want to either. However, most times we can really learn some important information by going back and recapturing what was happening for you at that time. Part of what I hope we can do together is enhance your ability to tolerate upsetting feelings—as you will be faced with future upsetting situations as a normal part of life.

TEEN: I'm feeling so much better now ...

THERAPIST: Sometimes the best time to discuss past problems is when you are feeling better. It can be a good time to look back and identify contributing factors and gain perspective that will help you look forward so that you can prevent future suicide attempts. This is one way to help you stay feeling good.

TEEN: I learned my lesson, so what's the point of dredging it up again?

THERAPIST: Good question, what is the point of dredging it up again? Well, the main point is that by better understanding everything that went on that day, you will have an increased sense of control when life is difficult. We will help you feel in control of "it" instead of "it" controlling you. What do you think about that?

Once the therapist has the teen's permission to move forward with the chain analysis, it is important to provide a further rationale for the exercise. For example:

"I am glad to hear that you are willing to tell your story. I think this will really help us get on the same page. I wonder if together we can try and identify all the factors (both external and internal) that possibly led to the attempt [or other problematic behavior]. Clearly, something was different about that day. If we can learn about all the contributing vulnerability factors, then we can identify strategies and skills for helping you anticipate, prepare for, and respond to, challenging life experiences."

HOW TO CONDUCT THE CHAIN ANALYSIS

The first step is to ask the adolescent (and later, the parents) to reconstruct the internal and external events leading up to the suicide attempt. To start, the therapist can ask the teen to walk him or her through the external events of the day (sometimes it may span more than one day) aloud. The therapist can ask, "Looking back, when do you think things started to go downhill?" Useful metaphors, such as watching a movie of the events that day (as in the freeze frame method), are helpful in conducting the chain analysis:

"I'd like for you to describe for me what was going on that day. If it is okay with you, I will write while you talk, so we can really *see* the day as it happened. By writing out the chain of events, we can identify key links in the chain of events that led to the attempt. Our goal is to re-create that day in so much detail that it is like we are watching a movie of the events of that day. By doing it this way, we can actually 'pause the movie' and identify critical 'scenes.'"

As the story progresses, the therapist can help the teen recall more detail by asking about relevant external and internal factors (e.g., where were you, who else was there, what were you doing, what were you thinking and feeling at each relevant point). The therapist can also heighten recall by asking more specific and concrete orienting questions, for example: "What was the weather like that day?" or "What were you wearing?" The therapist should also ask about any possible vulnerability factors that may have increased the likelihood that the attempt would occur on that day, rather than some other day. Some examples of vulnerability factors include fatigue, not getting enough sleep, substance use, caffeine use, and hormonal factors.

Included within the chain of events are the consequences and environmental responses to the problematic behavior. The therapist should inquire about specific consequences and responses, differentiating between short- and long-term consequences. For example, "After you took all the pills and went to the hospital, what happened next? How did people treat you in the hospital? How did your family react? What about your friends?" All of this information should be recorded on a chain analysis template (Figure 5.2).

CONDUCTING THE CHAIN ANALYSIS WITH PARENTS

After completing the chain analysis with the adolescent, we also recommend that the therapist review the chain of events with the teen's parents. Often times the parents have additional information, as well as a different perspective that is helpful for informing the approach to treatment. The method for conducting the chain analysis with the parents is the same as it is with the teen. The therapist can begin by asking the parents to share their experience of the event.

In some cases, the family may be reluctant to discuss the suicide attempt (or other problem behavior). The family may minimize the

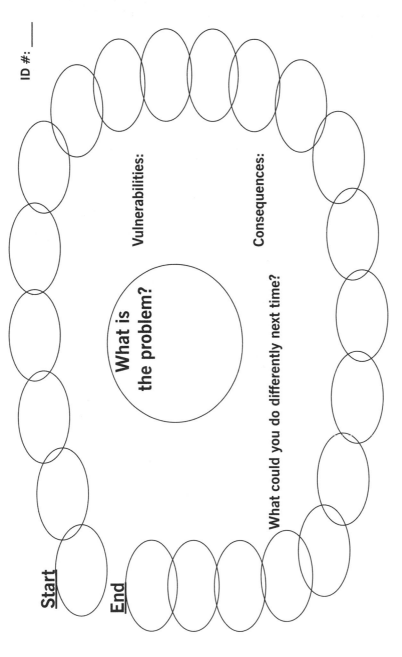

FIGURE 5.2. Chain analysis.

severity of the problem, or see the behavior as attention-seeking or manipulative. Some parents may be fearful that talking about the suicide attempt may make things worse. Other parents may see the behavior as "normal teenage behavior."

When faced with parental reluctance, it is important for the therapist to listen carefully to their point of view. The therapist needs to maintain a nonjudgmental approach with parents, as well as with their teens. Just as adolescents engage in behaviors for good reasons, so do parents. We often discover parents' fear that "the system" may blame them or identify them as solely responsible for their child's problems. In approaching the family, the therapist should remember that there may be multiple familial factors at play (e.g., parental mood disorders, intergenerational trauma, domestic violence, and/or environmental stressors), and that it is unlikely that any single event or risk factor can completely account for the suicide attempt.

ADDRESSING VULNERABILITY AND PROTECTIVE FACTORS

From the information yielded during conduct of the chain analysis, the therapist and teen will learn about important factors that contributed to the suicidal behavior. This information directly informs how the treatment should proceed. The therapist can introduce this approach to the adolescent by posing the following questions:

- "What was different that day?"
- "What made it more likely that you would engage in suicidal behavior [or other problem behavior] on that day, not on the day before?"

The therapist can follow up by explaining the rationale for trying to uncover the vulnerability factors that may have led up to and contributed to the problem behavior. Often, vulnerability factors are among the most amenable to change in therapy over a relatively short period of time. This is the case because vulnerability factors such as poor sleep habits are often tangible behaviors that the teen can easily recognize as being related to the problem behavior. Additionally, discussion of vulnerability factors tends to be less emotionally charged than discussion of some of the other related factors, such as interpersonal conflict. Thus, teens are more willing to address the vulnerability factors as opposed to other more emotionally charged topics (e.g., abuse, family conflict) early in treatment.

The chain analysis can also help to identify protective factors at work for the adolescent—that is, those factors that have helped to protect against risk. For example, the presence of a prosocial peer group, involvement in meaningful, proactive community or school activities, and connection with a supportive adult role model may help the adolescent to refrain from engaging in problem behaviors on other occasions.

The idea of addressing both vulnerability and protective factors in treatment is in line with recent research attempting to determine whether "compensation" or "capitalization" models of treatment are superior for the treatment of depression and suicidality. A compensation model (i.e., emphasis on vulnerability factors) focuses on remediating an individual's areas of relative weakness, whereas a capitalization model focuses on enhancing the individual's strengths. It remains largely unknown which of these approaches is more beneficial. The work that has been done thus far indicates that the type and extent of deficits may be critical to determining the optimal approach; some deficits are more amenable to change than others. For example, when problem-solving deficits are evident, a compensatory approach focusing on enhancing these skills appears to be effective, whereas social skills deficits may be slower to respond to skills training, and thus a capitalization model is preferable under these circumstances. Given the remaining questions in this area, we recommend that therapists take an inclusive approach in which both vulnerability factors and protective factors are addressed.

Vulnerability Factors

Vulnerability factors contribute to the teen's depression and to suicidal behavior. The failure to get sufficient sleep is one of the most significant factors that increases a teen's vulnerability to negative affect and risky behavior. Therefore, it is important to educate the teen early in treatment about how vulnerability factors like sleep problems affect mood and behavior. For example, most teens can easily identify that they are quicker to become annoyed or upset when sleep-deprived. The therapist can then coach the teen on the importance of developing good sleep habits. Suggestions for good sleep habits are presented in Figure 5.3.

In addition to developing good sleep habits, there are other strategies for decreasing vulnerability factors that can help teens to manage their emotions more effectively. We encourage teens to take care of

- Establish a regular time for going to bed and getting up in the morning, and stick to it even on weekends and vacations.
- Avoid naps during the day, even if you feel very tired.
- Avoid caffeine and nicotine, especially 4–6 hours before bedtime.
- Exercise regularly; however avoid exercise 4–6 hours before bedtime.
- Avoid drinking fluids just before bedtime, so that sleep is not disturbed by the need to use the bathroom.
- Avoid eating a large meal before bedtime. However, a light, soothing snack might help sleep.
- Use your bed for sleep only. Avoid reading, doing homework, or watching television in bed.
- Make sure your bed is comfortable and your room is quiet and a comfortable temperature.
- Take a hot bath about 1 hour before bedtime. The body temperature then begins dropping rapidly, which may aid sleep after that time (taking a bath shortly before bed actually increases alertness).
- Outside of bed, do something relaxing in the half-hour before bedtime. For example, read, listen to relaxing music, or do relaxation exercises.
- Do not look at the clock. Obsessing about the time will just make it more difficult to sleep.
- If you can't fall asleep within 15–20 minutes, get out of bed, go into another room, read, or try another quiet activity until you are sleepy again.

FIGURE 5.3. Suggestions for improving sleep.

other basic needs, such as engaging in regular eating habits. To illustrate, many teens will be able to recall a time when eating too much or too little had a negative impact on health, self-esteem, and mood.

We also encourage teens to exercise regularly. For teens who are not getting any exercise, it is important to start small and work toward a reasonable daily goal for that individual. Goals should take into account the teen's current physical health as well as previous levels of activity before onset of the depression. It is also important for the teen to strive for and maintain overall good physical health for, as we know, any physical illness or pain can impact emotional wellness.

It is essential to discuss with teens the role of drugs and alcohol in depressed mood and suicidality. Substance use can be a major contributor toward feeling depressed and out of control, and certainly impairs a teen's ability to make good decisions. Depressed teens who use alcohol or drugs are at greater risk for suicidal behavior.

Protective Factors

Many suicide attempters exhibit some ambivalence about wanting to die. Often when pressed, suicidal individuals can identify some part of themselves—no matter how small—that wants to live for a particular reason. This is where a therapist can work with a teen to identify and bolster factors that can be protective against self-destructive behavior.

There are two ways to identify protective factors. The first includes the specific things in a person's life that he or she may offer as "reasons for living." These may be either short- or long-term aspirations. For example, the teen may be looking forward to going to the prom, graduating from high school, having his or her own apartment, or getting married. The therapist should encourage the teen to elaborate on these future aims, and listen for any indication of hopelessness about reaching these goals. Rather than attributing their current distress to symptoms of an acute illness, many teens who are acutely depressed believe that they will always feel this way. The therapist should help the teen understand how specific symptoms of depression (e.g., hopelessness, declining motivation, anhedonia) may be contributing to the belief that future goals are unattainable. When the treatable illness improves, the teen will see his or her future differently. In this way, the therapist aims to build hopefulness about the future. The therapist can also ask specifically about what additional things have kept the teen from engaging in suicidal behavior. Some areas to explore include the teen's religious beliefs, connection to family members, friends, and pets, and commitments to future plans.

The second way to incorporate protective factors into treatment comes to us from the current literature. Research on depressed teens consistently supports the idea that certain factors in a teen's life can help guard against suicide. These include affiliation with a healthy, prosocial peer group, connection to school and community, and active engagement with family. The therapist may attempt to increase protective factors for the teen by facilitating increased involvement in these three important areas. For example:

> THERAPIST: So, I know everyone in your family is so very busy, and this makes it very hard for you to spend time all together.
>
> MOM: Yeah, I am working two jobs, and Joey's got football practice four nights per week. I am also running back and forth picking up the baby from daycare. It's all I can do to keep up.
>
> THERAPIST: Absolutely. You have a lot going on. When do you and Joey see each other?

JOEY: We don't really.

MOM: Yeah, he's right. We barely see each other but for a short time in the morning ...

THERAPIST: It sounds like life is really getting in the way of you spending time together. Is that something you wish could be different?

JOEY: Yes, we used to talk all the time before the baby came along.

MOM: I miss those times, but I just can't do any more than I'm doing.

THERAPIST: I get that you are maxed out, and with the baby, things aren't the same. But I wonder if there is any way we can find a little time like you used to have.

MOM: That would be good—I just don't see when.

JOEY: What about in the morning ... when the baby is still sleeping? Maybe we could at least eat at the same time.

MOM: That's a good idea, but the morning seems so rushed.

THERAPIST: Um, so what would it take to make this work?

MOM: Well, maybe if we got up 5 or 10 minutes earlier?

THERAPIST: That sounds good—what do you think, Joey?

JOEY: I think we should try it.

THERAPIST: Great, can't wait to hear how it goes.

The basic premise involved in addressing vulnerability and protective factors is that by attending to the basics of life, we can all enhance our ability to effectively manage daily life stressors and strong emotions, because we are less vulnerable and more protected from their effects.

TREATMENT PLANNING

Collaborative Development of the Treatment Plan

The process for developing a treatment plan with the patient and family should be collaborative. There are three reasons why a collaborative approach is important. First, it is important for the teen and family to feel in charge of the treatment, since they are the ones who will implement the treatment decisions. Families who feel coerced into a treatment program usually will not follow through. Second, there are often several approaches that all have more or less equivalent support; if the patient and family feel strongly about one of those options, and the therapist is competent to implement it, then that option represents a reasonable place to start. The therapist should present what is known about different treatment options, including their advantages and disadvantages, and then work with the teen and family to select options that the therapist thinks will help and that the patient and family can endorse. Third, despite the contribution of several important research studies, the complexity of many of our patients poses clinical questions that go beyond the results of clinical trials. This means that our treatment plans are based on a combination of the extant literature and clinical experience, and that taking an authoritarian stance often cannot be supported empirically.

How to Create a Treatment Plan

Once the teen and therapist have mapped out the sequence of events and other pertinent details about the suicide attempt using the chain analysis, and incorporated the family's input, we use the chain to collaboratively develop the plan for treatment. To begin, the teen and therapist look closely at the chain to find the critical points. We sometimes use the analogy of "playing detective." That is, we look carefully at the case for clues to make sense of what happened and why. This is done by paying close attention to the weak links in the chain. In other words, any relative skill deficits (e.g., poor distress tolerance, limited problem-solving ability, and/or self-critical cognitive style) may be identified as potential treatment targets. For example:

> "How about if you and I look carefully at the chain and try to identify any areas that we think could have been critical links leading up to the suicide attempt? This will help us begin to create a treatment plan. It is important for us to pay special attention to the interventions that will do the most to diminish your risk for another attempt. Once you and I have agreed on what we think is important to work on, I was thinking we could meet with your parents to get their input and agree on a treatment plan. How does that sound?"

After the specific proximal risk factors have been noted, the therapist and teen should determine which problems or skills deficits are perceived to be the most life-threatening or dangerous. Often, there are many different therapeutic strategies that could be a focus of treatment. The prioritization of specific skills should focus on those skills that are most likely to prevent a subsequent suicide attempt (or other high-priority problem behavior). The most dangerous problems or skill deficits may be more apparent if the problems or skill deficits occurred during events leading to previous attempts. The selection of the specific therapeutic interventions should be determined by the teen and therapist together. As can be seen on the treatment planning form (Figure 5.4), several questions help us to choose a specific intervention strategy:

1. Which intervention is perceived by *both* the therapist and patient to be the *most helpful* for preventing suicidal behavior?
2. Which intervention would have helped to make a difference in preventing a previous attempt?
3. Which intervention builds upon the *existing strengths and resources* of the patient?
4. Which intervention is the patient willing to undertake?

In addition to discussions with the teen about possible intervention choices, the teen's family should be consulted. The treatment plan may certainly be updated as new information about the proximal risk and protective factors are revealed, or when additional information is obtained that further informs the plan.

Prioritization in the Face of Multiple Problems

Problems should be prioritized in the following order: those that are life-threatening, those that threaten the therapy, and then those symptoms or disorders that are the most functionally impairing. Life-threatening behavior, like suicidal or homicidal behavior, intravenous drug use, or nonadherence to treatment for a chronic illness (e.g., insulin for diabetics), should be addressed even before the depression, even if depression is contributing to the problem. Therapy-threatening issues, like the parent or adolescent not agreeing with the treatment plan, feeling hopeless about treatment, or simply living too far from the therapist to be able to come routinely for treatment, should all be addressed prior to developing an extensive treatment plan. Since depressed youth frequently present with comorbid disorders, the symptoms that are causing the greatest functional impairment should be addressed first. Comorbid conditions should also be targeted first if the successful treatment of depression is predicated on proper management of the comorbid condition. A depressed teen with anorexia who is nutritionally compromised should have her nutritional status normalized prior to treating her depression. On the other hand, a normal-weight teen with bulimia whose bingeing seems related to negative affect and poor self-esteem may actually need

Problem	Related Vulnerability Factors	Related Protective Factors	Intervention(s) Most Likely to Target the Problem (*circle*)	Barriers to Implementation
1.			Behavioral activation Emotion regulation Cognitive restructuring Interpersonal effectiveness Distress tolerance Other	
2.			Behavioral activation Emotion regulation Cognitive restructuring Interpersonal effectiveness Distress tolerance Other	
3.			Behavioral activation Emotion regulation Cognitive restructuring Interpersonal effectiveness Distress tolerance Other	

FIGURE 5.4. Treatment planning form.

to have the depression treated in order to effectively resolve the eating disorder. An adolescent with depression and opiate dependence should be detoxified and in treatment for substance abuse prior to any attempt to treat the depression, whereas a youth who has a clear depressive episode antedating binge drinking may benefit from simultaneous management of the depression and alcohol use. A patient with comorbid depression and ADHD who is suicidal, socially withdrawn, and hopeless should probably have the depression as the first treatment priority, whereas a patient whose depression is secondary to school failure and peer rejection because of impulsivity might best have the ADHD treated first.

Presenting the Treatment Plan to the Family

The therapist and the teen can present their ideas for treatment to the family and invite the parents to provide input and feedback. Specific treatment targets should be agreed upon by the entire family. This is also an ideal opportunity to discuss and agree on the frequency of sessions, as well as the balance between individual and family sessions.

CASE EXAMPLE

Joe was a 17-year-old who had been a star soccer player. After his girlfriend broke up with him several months ago, he started to withdraw socially, and his grades started slipping. When he became ineligible to play soccer due to his poor GPA, he made a suicide attempt. Chain analysis revealed that after Joe's girlfriend broke up with him, he experienced an acute drop in mood, difficulty concentrating in school, and hopelessness about his future. The breakup, coupled with declining grades and removal from the soccer team, resulted in a significant decrease in Joe's self-esteem. Joe claimed that prior to this year, things had generally been pretty easy for him, and so he simply felt he could not cope when the multiple stressors came along. As a result, Joe and his therapist collaborated on a preliminary plan for treatment that would help enhance his problem-solving and distress tolerance skills. Once this agreement was made, they agreed to invite his parents into the session to present the plan and get their feedback.

> THERAPIST: Thanks for coming in tonight. Joe and I had a very productive session and came up with some ideas for treatment we would like to share with you.
>
> MOM: OK. We are curious to hear what you came up with. We want to be sure this never happens again.

THERAPIST: Joe, how about if you start off by letting your parents know about how we have come to understand what led to your suicide attempt, and how we are thinking about approaching treatment.

JOE: I guess I can start. So I realized that up until lately, things kind of came easy for me. I mean, I always did pretty well in school and sports, and have been pretty lucky when it came to my friends and girlfriends and stuff. So when Meg broke up with me and I didn't see it coming, it hit me pretty hard. And since I never really had to deal with anything like that before, I just didn't know what to do or how to handle it. So we were thinking that maybe we'd work on finding me some other ways to handle it when tough things happen. 'Cause as much as I hate to admit it, I could probably use some help in that area.

DAD: That makes sense to me.

MOM: Me too.

Therapist: Thanks, Joe. You did a great job summarizing for your parents our thoughts about where to go with treatment. Mr. and Mrs. Jones, how does that plan sound to you?

MOM: Really good. Although I would love it if life was always easy for Joe, let's face it, bad things can happen. And I'd like to see him be able to handle it when they do.

DAD: Me too.

THERAPIST: OK, so it sounds like we are all in agreement that we are headed in the right direction here. Anything else that will be important for Joe and me to focus on from your perspectives?

MOM: Nothing that I can think of.

DAD: Me neither.

INTEGRATED CASE EXAMPLE

Throughout this chapter, we have described the process for getting from assessment of the suicidal behavior using chain analysis to collaboratively formulating the treatment plan. We conclude with one integrated case example that illustrates how these components come together in clinical practice.

Martha was a 16-year-old who took a nearly lethal overdose of Tylenol. She and her boyfriend, Brian, were at a party and she had been drinking. They began to fight at the party after Martha saw Brian talking to another girl. Martha left the party, walked home, and took the pills. Her motivation was to get her boyfriend to feel guilty and sorry and to pay more attention to her; she did not care if she lived or died.

Martha was in a depressive episode and also had significant anxiety. She reported that Brian was her best friend, and that she counted on him for "everything," which he found "too intense." Before her involvement with him, she spent time with a couple of good female friends and was active in the marching band and her church youth group. Since the onset of her depression, Martha reported that she had lost motivation for these activities. Additionally, she found she didn't have time to both do these things and maintain a relationship with Brian.

Martha and her therapist worked on a chain analysis (see Figure 5.5) of the suicide attempt:

THERAPIST: What do you think set this off?

MARTHA: My boyfriend and I got into a fight about him talking so much to Susie. He said I was too clingy; I said if he really loved

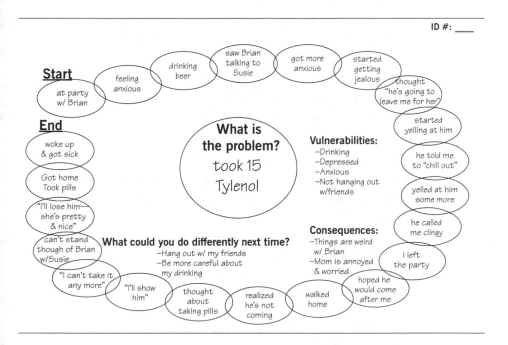

FIGURE 5.5. Sample chain analysis for Martha.

me, he would want to spend time with me, not Susie ... and it just got worse from there.

THERAPIST: What happened then?

MARTHA: I took off.

THERAPIST: OK. What were you thinking and feeling at that point?

MARTHA: I was really angry and hoping he would come after me to apologize. Once I saw he wasn't going to leave the party, I thought, I'll show him.

THERAPIST: Anything else?

MARTHA: I can't live without Brian. I don't feel good without him. I couldn't stand the thought of him being with Susie—I know she likes him.

THERAPIST: Was there anything else going on at this point that tipped you in the direction of a suicide attempt?

MARTHA: Well, I have not been feeling that great lately. I feel kinda "blah" and nervous all the time, and it was really getting hard to take.

THERAPIST: Right, but what made it different right then?

MARTHA: Maybe it was worse because we had the fight and I started thinking I would lose him to Susie. She's so pretty and everyone likes her.

THERAPIST: Was there anything else different for you that night?

MARTHA: I drank more than usual ...

THERAPIST: Can you tell me about that?

MARTHA: I think I had around four or five beers at the party.

THERAPIST: And how were you feeling?

MARTHA: At first, I had a good buzz and felt more comfortable and outgoing. But then I started to get jealous and couldn't keep it to myself.

THERAPIST: So, then what happened?

MARTHA: While he was busy with Susie, I started yelling at him. And then he told me to chill out. That made me more mad. All I wanted was for him to stop talking to her and pay attention to me.

THERAPIST: You said you wanted to get him to pay more attention to you. So, did he?

MARTHA: No, not then. So, I just left, hoping he would follow; but he didn't.

THERAPIST: So, when did you first have the thought of taking the pills?

MARTHA: As I was walking home. As soon as I realized he wasn't coming after me, I felt real bad, and thought I would show him.

THERAPIST: Once you got home, what happened from there?

MARTHA: My mom and dad were sleeping. So, I just went upstairs to the bathroom medicine cabinet and found a bottle of Tylenol. I think I took 15 or so and went to bed.

THERAPIST: What were you hoping would happen?

MARTHA: I didn't really care if I lived or died. I just couldn't take it anymore. One part of me was hoping he would call or text me, so I kept checking my phone. The other part of me just didn't care.

THERAPIST: So, then what happened?

MARTHA: A couple hours later, I woke up feeling really sick. While I was in the bathroom throwing up, my mom came in to check on me. She asked me what happened, and I told her about the Tylenol.

THERAPIST: How did your mom react?

MARTHA: She was real worried and seemed a little mad too. She woke my dad and they took me to the emergency room. The doctor at the hospital said I would be OK and sent me to see you.

THERAPIST: OK. And what happened with Brian?

MARTHA: Well, he called me the next day. I told him what happened and he felt really bad and apologized. Things are OK with us now, but still a little weird.

THERAPIST: Martha, we know people do things for very good reasons. It sounds like a lot was going on for you that night. Could we look at the "links" in the chain together and try to really understand what led you to take the pills? This will help us figure out what may have been some of the key factors involved and how we can work on them in treatment so that we can decrease the chances this will ever happen again.

MARTHA: Yeah, I guess.

THERAPIST: So, it seems like you have been feeling depressed and anxious lately. Also, since you started dating Brian, it seems like you haven't had the time to see your other friends as much. So, it makes sense that once you got to the party, you started drinking to try and feel more social. Then you saw Susie talking to Brian, which was a huge trigger for you. It seems like this really set off a bunch of worried thoughts. Am I getting it right?

MARTHA: Yes, exactly—and it all seemed to happen so quickly.

THERAPIST: The other thing I noticed in looking at the chain is how intense the emotions are for you, and how hard it is when you are upset to communicate what you really need.

MARTHA: Yes, I don't think people get how intense my emotions are. Brian says I am way too emotional, and I guess he is kinda right—I shouldn't need him so much.

THERAPIST: So, I am thinking maybe we could work together on helping you feel more in control of your own emotions. Then we could work on identifying what emotional needs you may have, being OK with those needs, and exploring how to express these needs to others in a way they can hear.

MARTHA: Yes, I agree with those ideas. I really don't want this kind of thing to ever happen again—it was all so terrible. Also, I just heard from my friend that Brian is really tired of all this drama. I can kind of tell underneath that things aren't that good with us.

THERAPIST: Are there other things you noticed from the chain that we might spend some time talking about?

MARTHA: Well, I guess I realized I felt alone at the party. Since I stopped hanging out with my girlfriends, I don't have anyone to talk to, other than Brian. I used to be in band and church youth group, but it seemed to take up so much time.

THERAPIST: Were these things that made you feel good in the past?

MARTHA: Yes, they did.

THERAPIST: Well, does it make sense for us to see how you could build some things back into your life, without overdoing it?

MARTHA: Yeah, I would like to.

THERAPIST: Great, maybe we could start there and come up with something small you could try this week to get hooked back in with your friends?

MARTHA: Great idea.

THERAPIST: So, we covered a lot of ground today, and you did a great job. We have some good ideas about where to go from here. How would you feel about us sharing our ideas with your parents?

MARTHA: OK, that would probably make them feel better; they have been very worried about me.

The case example above demonstrates how the therapist and teen collaboratively go through the chain analysis of a suicide attempt and identify priorities for intervention.

KEY POINTS

- A chain analysis is a detailed functional analysis of any behavior.
- Conducting the chain analysis allows the therapist and teen to develop a better understanding of the function of the suicidal behavior (or other problem behavior).
- It is important to clearly discuss the rationale for the chain analysis with the teen before attempting the exercise.
- The chain analysis should involve detailed review of events, thoughts, feelings, and vulnerability and protective factors, as well as the consequences of the behavior.
- Once the chain analysis is complete, the therapist and teen can use the information to determine what needs the suicidal behavior was intended to meet, and identify which skills would be most beneficial to focus on in treatment.
- When the therapist and teen are prioritizing among multiple problems contributing to the suicidal behavior, those that are most closely linked to repeated suicidal behavior, as well as those most likely to be effective, should be focused on first in treatment.

CHAPTER 6

Behavioral Activation and Emotion Regulation

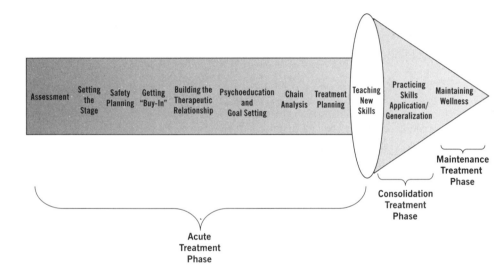

WHAT YOU WILL LEARN IN THIS CHAPTER

- What behavioral activation is.
- When to implement behavioral activation with a depressed adolescent.
- How to conduct behavioral activation with an adolescent.
- What emotion regulation skills are.
- How to teach some basic emotion regulation skills to teens and families, including:
  - ◆ Education about emotions.
  - ◆ Acceptance of emotion.
  - ◆ The emotions thermometer.

♦ Distraction.

♦ Deep breathing.

A fundamental principle of the cognitive model of depression is that thoughts, feelings, and behaviors are interconnected. Studies have shown that the therapist can intervene at any point in the depressive spiral, because altering any of these components of depression will have an effect on the other two. In this chapter, we focus on two of these components: actions and emotions. Interventions that encourage positive activity are termed *behavioral activation*. Interventions that directly target negative emotions are termed *emotion regulation*. The therapist may choose one or both of these approaches, either because a major source of the patient's difficulties is lack of activity or difficulty with emotion regulation, or because the patient may be more receptive to these interventions than to some alternative approaches.

BEHAVIORAL ACTIVATION

Behavioral activation involves encouraging the teen to engage in behavior that is ordinarily reinforcing and enjoyable, and will enhance the patient's sense of mastery, accomplishment, and self-esteem. Improvements in mood have been shown to be linked to increased engagement in such activities.

Depressive symptoms such as decreased ability to experience pleasure and loss of energy or motivation can cause the depressed teen to disengage from activities that he or she formerly found rewarding, such as socializing with friends, participating in sports, or other activities. Withdrawal from these activities may further contribute to worsening of other symptoms of depression. For example, a depressed teen who turns down offers to socialize with friends may find that his or her friends eventually stop calling. This may lead the teen to feel abandoned by them. Spending time alone allows for rumination and sadness, due to both the lack of distracting activities and the absence of positive reinforcement. We all need to experience a sense of accomplishment—which is hard to do if one is inactive and disengaged.

We therefore set the stage for behavioral activation by explaining to teens that as long as they remain withdrawn and disengaged, the likelihood of experiencing positive emotions is very low. By "getting active," even if at first they do not experience any mood improvement, they create the *possibility* of feeling better.

For Whom Are These Interventions Likely to Be Helpful?

Teens who have become highly inactive and withdrawn, those who lack structure, and those who have few sources of positive affect in their lives benefit from behavioral activation. Additionally, compared to other components of CBT, behavioral activation may be more helpful for youth who have difficulty identifying emotions and monitoring their thoughts. Finally, some depressed teens may not be able to benefit from other aspects of therapy until their mood begins to lift. Behavioral activation is the fastest, most intuitive method for helping reverse depressive symptoms.

The objective of behavioral activation is to help the teen structure his or her time to engage in pleasurable and meaningful activities. We now describe a step-by-step approach to the implementation of behavioral activation with depressed teens.

Assessment of Current Activities

The first step in behavioral activation is to learn what the depressed teen's schedule looks like right now. Each activity can then be rated on a scale of 1–5 (1 being the least, 5 the most) with respect to pleasure ("How enjoyable was this") and mastery ("To what extent did you feel a sense of accomplishment?"). The patient should also rate his or her mood and suicidality during those times. On the basis of this review, the therapist and patient can identify whether there are activities and/ or times of day that are particularly helpful or problematic.

Here is an example of a patient, Judd, age 16, who has identified an activity as being helpful to his mood but often does not feel like doing it:

> THERAPIST: You said that on Thursday afternoon you went for a run and seemed to enjoy it. On some of the other afternoons you reported not doing too much, and it seemed like those were the days your mood was pretty low.
>
> JUDD: Yes, that's true. When I exercise, I definitely feel better and feel better about myself. But lots of days I don't feel like doing it.
>
> THERAPIST: What do you think happens first? Do you feel better and then go running, or do you run and then feel better?
>
> JUDD: Definitely the second. I was not feeling so good on Thursday but just got it into my head to go running.

Inventory of Past Enjoyable Activities

Often depressed teens will completely stop participating in the activities they once found enjoyable. In such instances, the therapist should try to find out which activities were enjoyable in the past. Choosing behavioral activation strategies involves not only selecting what *is* likely to work, but also avoiding what is *not* likely to work. In the example that follows, we take a look at an activity that seems likely to enhance the patient's mood.

THERAPIST: Ginny, I know that you are not finding much of anything fun lately since your depression has gotten worse. A few weeks ago you even stopped going to dance class, which I know you used to really like.

GINNY: Yeah, I just don't see the point. I mean, I know I am not going to be able to get into it like I used to.

THERAPIST: Right. Your depression has made it much harder to enjoy things.

GINNY: Yeah, I guess.

THERAPIST: How did you use to feel during and after dance class?

GINNY: I felt good because I caught on pretty fast, and sometimes the teacher would even have me demonstrate for the rest of the class. That was pretty cool.

THERAPIST: Absolutely. Sounds like going to dance class made you feel like you were good at something.

GINNY: Yeah.

THERAPIST: So, the last few Tuesday nights—what have you been doing instead of going to dance class?

GINNY: Nothing really.

THERAPIST: And how has your mood been on those Tuesdays?

GINNY: Pretty down—just like always. I usually just lay around the house.

THERAPIST: Would you say that resting at home on Tuesdays is not helping you feel any better?

GINNY: No, not really. I just feel the same. Kinda sad and down.

THERAPIST: So, what are the chances that this week staying home on Tuesday will help you feel better?

GINNY: Like, none.

THERAPIST: Here's what I am thinking: that even though you are not motivated to go to dance class now, and you expect that you won't be able to get into it like before, I am wondering if there's any chance that you might feel even a bit better if you went.

GINNY: Maybe.

Now, we take a look at an activity that a depressed teen might choose to postpone or modify in some way.

THERAPIST: So, tell me, what were some of the things you really enjoyed doing that gave you a sense of accomplishment?

MOLLY: I was editor of my school newspaper. I really liked being at the center of things, and it was cool to see how it came together every month.

THERAPIST: And what made you stop doing it?

MOLLY: In order to get the paper out on time, we often had to pull all-nighters. I can barely stay awake at school these days when I get 10 hours of sleep. I just don't think I could go without sleep. I am also having a hard time thinking clearly. When I was the editor, I had to make a lot of big decisions.

THERAPIST: It sounds like, while being involved as editor was really rewarding, it was also demanding. Maybe now is not the best time for you to pick that back up. Is there something else related to the newspaper that you could do that might be meaningful?

MOLLY: Well, I like to write. I could work on some features that don't have such a tight deadline and leave the editing head-aches to someone else.

Generating a List of Possible Activities

Teens who are highly inactive and those who initially have difficulty identifying any pleasurable activities often require an activity schedule to counter the inertia of depression. To begin, the therapist and the teen should work together to generate a list of at least 10 activities that the teen may find enjoyable. If the teen has difficulty generating any pleasant activities, the therapist can inquire about activities that the teen *used* to find enjoyable before he or she became depressed. With the teen, keep in mind the following guidelines for scheduling pleasant activities. Ideal activities are those that:

1. Can be done easily and frequently (e.g., a teen who has never ice-skated should not start with joining an ice hockey team).
2. Do not cost a lot of money.
3. Have a social aspect.
4. Are likely to increase well-being and sense of accomplishment.

Activity Scheduling

After reviewing the list of new activities, as well as activities that the patient formerly enjoyed, the therapist and teen can look at his or her current schedule (see Figure 6.1) and determine which activities could be added. For each activity, it is useful for the teen and therapist to consider what the payoff might be, as well as the possible barriers that might get in the way of doing a particular activity. The therapist should encourage the teen to begin with activities that are easy to do and likely to provide short-term reinforcement.

The therapist should emphasize to the depressed teen that one can plan and engage in such activities—and derive benefit—*even when one does not feel like it.* In fact, the therapist may specifically encourage the teen to separate feelings from behavior. Indeed, sometimes people must act in ways that are not consistent with how they feel in order to achieve goals; hopefully the teen will also experience improved mood in the process. We will continue with the example of Judd:

THERAPIST: Since you have noticed your mood is better on days when you run, what would it be like for you to try scheduling a daily run?

JUDD: Even if I don't feel like it?

THERAPIST: *Especially* if you don't feel like it! Oftentimes depression can make you feel like you don't want to do things, even though doing those things can help you feel better.

Together, the therapist and teen can identify those activities on the list they will focus on in the coming week, and can discuss specific days and times when the teen will engage in specific behaviors. Together, the therapist and teen can set goals for the number of activities the teen will engage in between sessions (e.g., one per day). The therapist may also ask the teen to rate his or her mood before as well as after the activity; the goal is to draw links between the teen's mood and engaging in specific activities. The teen should be encouraged to test out if a particular activity is beneficial or not. He or she can then decide whether to continue the activity.

Time	Monday	Tuesday	Wednesday	Thursday	Friday	Saturday	Sunday
8–9							
9–10							
10–11							
11–12							
12–1							
1–2							
2–3							
3–4							
4–5							
5–6							
6–7							
7–8							
8–9							
9–10							
10–11							

FIGURE 6.1. Daily diary.

At times, the therapist may find it helpful to break down certain scheduled activities into smaller, more attainable components. To illustrate:

THERAPIST: So, Rob, you have written on the activity schedule that you'd like to aim to do your homework from 4 to 6 o'clock on weekdays.

ROB: Yes.

THERAPIST: I know that you are taking many challenging classes right now and often feel like you have a ton of homework.

ROB: Right. I get pretty overwhelmed by it.

THERAPIST: I can see why! I am wondering if it would help for us to think specifically about how you can best use those 2 hours you would like to schedule for homework?

ROB: Definitely. Sometimes even when I have enough time to finish it, I can't figure out where to start.

THERAPIST: OK. So, what about if we break it down by course?

ROB: That makes sense. So, I have algebra, biology, and English class on Monday, Wednesday, and Friday. So, I should probably schedule homework time for those three classes on Sunday, Tuesday, and Thursday afternoons. Then for Spanish class I have a vocabulary quiz every Thursday. So, let's put studying for my Spanish quiz on Wednesday night's schedule. And I don't have any homework for gym class. The last one is my history class. I have that class on Tuesday and Thursday, and usually have a chapter to read to prepare. So, I guess that goes on Monday and Wednesday nights' schedule.

THERAPIST: Excellent, Rob! Can you see how getting more specific about how to use that homework time slot can be helpful to you?

ROB: Yes, when I think about it this way, it seems much easier. I can try it this week and see how it goes.

Family Involvement

Family members can be helpful in implementing behavioral activation strategies. While involvement in behavioral activation is a good idea in most families, it may be contraindicated for families in which there is a high level of discord or for adolescents who express a strong need for independence.

While the teen needs to take responsibility for implementing the activity, other family members may engage in pleasant activities with the teen. Family member involvement can both increase the likelihood that the teen will use the skill, and also contribute to positive family connections—a protective factor against depression and suicidality. Because behavioral activation is very concrete, it can be a particularly helpful skill for parents who report difficulty knowing what to say or do to help their teen feel better.

Families characterized by low cohesion may also benefit from this skill. The therapist can explain to families that when a family member becomes depressed, other members of the family may disengage from one another. The family therefore may benefit from scheduling time to engage in activities together. In Ginny's case, introduced earlier, the therapist might involve the family as follows:

THERAPIST: One of the things that we are working on with Ginny is helping her to increase her pleasant activities, especially when she is beginning to feel depressed. It is important to get Ginny active again and interacting with people more. She is working on some plans to do this, and we think it could be helpful if you would encourage this and support these activities. How would you feel about that?

DAD: OK, I think we can do that.

THERAPIST: Ginny had a couple ideas about possible activities she could plan to do. Ginny, would you like to tell your dad some of the ideas we came up with?

GINNY: Yeah, sure. I was thinking about asking Suzie to go to the movie this weekend. Remember how we used to do that and then we would shop at the mall?

DAD: Yes, you haven't gone out with Suzie in a long time.

THERAPIST: Dad, is there anything you could do to help with this plan?

DAD: Sure, I can take you and pick you up if you would like.

GINNY: That would be good, assuming Suzie can go.

THERAPIST: Great. This is a good start to our overall strategy for increasing Ginny's pleasant activities. Is there anything you used to enjoy doing with your family?

GINNY: We used to do a lot of things—but everyone seems so busy.

DAD: Yes, we are busy, but if we really tried, I think we could do some of the things we used to enjoy together.

GINNY: What about getting back to watching the football game on Sunday together like we used to?

DAD: Great idea, your mom would enjoy that too. I'll make the popcorn.

THERAPIST: Great idea, anything else?

DAD: Maybe you and your mother could start walking Big Ben [the dog] together after dinner?

GINNY: Maybe, while it's still nice outside.

THERAPIST: You both have come up with some very good ideas today. Clearly, one important step toward helping Ginny get well and stay well is to help her get active again. Anything the family can do to support her efforts would be very helpful.

This case example demonstrates how the therapist can encourage the family to discuss and choose pleasant activities they can enjoy together as a family. In addition, family members can support the teen's efforts to engage in activities with peers. The decision to include siblings in family activities should be based on the age of siblings and the quality of their preexisting relationship. Some additional examples of pleasant family activities include watching a movie together, attending a sporting event, going out to dinner, working out together, and playing a board game. As with any behavioral activation strategy, the plan should include the specifics of where and when. The therapist and family should consider possible barriers that might get in the way of the plan and should generate possible solutions.

EMOTION REGULATION

Emotion regulation skills are designed to help the teen handle strong emotions like anger or sadness. Strong emotions can lead to suffering and also cloud the teen's ability to think clearly and make effective choices. We describe two different approaches to managing strong emotions: (1) improving the ability to *tolerate* strong emotions (distress tolerance) and (2) improving the ability to *modulate* strong emotions (emotion regulation). As discussed in Chapter 2, trying to escape strong negative emotions is a common reason for engaging in suicidal behavior. Also, when depressed teens are overwhelmed with strong emotions, they are much less likely to effectively use problem-solving skills. As a result, they are more likely to select an impulsive and maladaptive solution to a perceived problem.

As with all skills that we introduce to the teen, we explain the rationale for the approach and get the teen's permission and support to discuss/work on the strategy. Please also see Bonner (2002) for additional information. The following case example illustrates how a therapist might get a teen on board with the idea of learning emotion regulation skills.

THERAPIST: Rick, we realized together last week when we reviewed your chain that it is hard for you to think clearly when you are experiencing strong emotions. I was thinking we could spend some time today and try to figure out some things that may help you when you are experiencing strong emotions like you did that day. What do you think about that?

RICK: But I'm feeling fine now. It's when I get upset that I need help.

THERAPIST: That's right! What is it that happened that day that got you so upset?

RICK: Well, my girlfriend told me she didn't want to see me anymore, and I felt so angry I couldn't stand it. That's why I made the attempt, to escape those feelings.

THERAPIST: Rick, you're exactly right! Most times when we are not upset, we do fine. It's when we feel those strong feelings that we have difficulty. I would love it if you never had to experience another difficult emotion again. How likely do you think that is?

RICK: Not likely.

THERAPIST: So, what about the idea of us working on a strategy now, while you are not distressed? That way the next time you feel that way, you will have some additional strategies for coping.

RICK: We can try.

The therapist can place the importance of emotion regulation skills in the context of overall therapeutic goals. Everyone has a more difficult time thinking clearly in the face of strong emotions—either negative (e.g., anger, frustration) or positive (early stage of romantic love). While emotion regulation skills will primarily help the teen learn to manage difficult emotions, they will also improve the teen's ability to effectively implement any other skills learned in treatment (e.g., communication skills). The therapist can begin by asking the teen to recall a time when he or she felt strong emotions. The therapist can then inquire about the details, including what made it hard for him or her to manage the emotions. The therapist can explain that emotion regulation skills help us to control our emotions rather than having our emotions control us.

As we have discussed throughout the book, before the therapist can teach and help the teen use any new skill, it is essential to first validate the teen's emotional experience (both currently and at the time of the suicide attempt). We illustrate again with Rick:

> THERAPIST: Let's go back to the day you had the fight with your girlfriend. You said you felt angry, right?
>
> RICK: I remember being angry—thinking, "You can't do this to me."
>
> THERAPIST: I can totally understand that. You clearly had every reason to feel that way. Under the circumstances, I think many people would have felt that way.
>
> RICK: Yes, I was also really embarrassed that she was dumping me and that everyone at school would know. I couldn't stand the thought of facing everyone on Monday.
>
> THERAPIST: Absolutely, I agree that would be very hard to deal with. Not only were you mad at her, but you also had to deal with feeling embarrassed. That's a lot of strong emotions to handle.

Notice that the therapist does not try to challenge the patient as to the appropriateness of any of his feelings, but simply validates their presence. Additionally, the therapist avoids the common pitfall of offering reassurance that his pain will pass and he will find another girlfriend. This case also illustrates that it is common for people to feel several emotions. Here, Rick was angry and also embarrassed.

Acceptance of Emotion

Many teens have the impression that certain emotions are "bad." In order for them to become more adept at regulating emotions, it is critical to help teens to accept their emotional experiences without judgment. The therapist can start by discussing with the teen any ideas he or she may have about bad or unacceptable emotions. How has the teen come to hold the idea that these emotions are bad? It can be helpful to distinguish between the emotion itself and the behavior that results from acting on an emotion.

Therapists can also help teens become aware of what they may say to themselves upon feeling strong emotions such as anger and sadness. That is, in addition to judging the emotion (e.g., good or bad), we may also judge ourselves for having the emotion (e.g., "I shouldn't feel this way"; "I am selfish for feeling this way"). Using a case example, we illustrate how self-judgment about emotions can compound emotional distress.

> THERAPIST: Can you think of a time you felt a really strong emotion?
>
> JOHN: Yes, I was really worked up earlier this week when I found out I was one point away from having an A in math.
>
> THERAPIST: OK, let's go with that example. I want you to try and recall how you felt when you first found out.
>
> JOHN: I was really upset.
>
> THERAPIST: OK. On a scale of 1–10, how upset were you when you first found out about your grade?
>
> JOHN: Maybe a 4.
>
> THERAPIST: OK. Now, can you try to recall what was going through your head once you found out your grade?
>
> JOHN: Hmmm ... well, first I was first thinking how unfair Mr. Jones was being. Then I realized how dumb I was for getting mad about it. I mean, other people get B's all the time and they don't get all upset. I shouldn't feel this way.
>
> THERAPIST: How upset are you feeling right now, as you recall those thoughts?
>
> JOHN: I still feel really mad at myself for being so upset about it ... like maybe a 7.
>
> THERAPIST: Right. Often, we can make an emotion feel even worse just by how we think about our feelings.

The therapist and teen can then explore additional feelings that are particularly difficult for the teen to manage. The aim is to help the teen to notice his or her emotional experience without judging him- or herself for feeling the emotion(s). A particularly important notion to highlight and discuss with teens is that "we are not our emotions." Although a teen may feel a certain emotion in the moment—for example, anger—this does not mean that he or she is "an angry person." Rather, he or she is feeling angry at that moment.

Education about Emotions

Emotions are not intrinsically good or bad. They can be thought of as signals about the importance and relevance of a given situation to a person. Fear is a signal that a situation is perceived as dangerous. Anger is experienced when a situation does not fit our expectations, such as when someone else is taking unfair advantage of us. Sadness occurs when a person loses something of value (material or interpersonal) or does not come up to his or her own expectations. Warmth, friendship, and love help to maintain important social bonds. For a given context, each of these emotions is appropriate and even adaptive. In fact, a person who does not experience fear in the face of a dangerous situation risks death or injury. Depressed and suicidal teens, as a general rule, have a lower threshold for experiencing emotions, and once an emotional response is triggered, they experience more intense and more prolonged emotions.

The therapist can explain to the teen that emotions serve multiple purposes. Emotions can be helpful and are often critical for survival. For example, our emotions help signal to us when something is wrong and also help us communicate with others. Together with the teen, the therapist can explore other ways in which emotions (even painful ones) have been helpful in his or her life. Some teens may have the belief that if they are effective and skillful, they will never experience another painful or unpleasant emotion. The therapist can have the teen imagine a world in which people did not have emotions. What would that be like?

> FRANK: I would rather be numb and just not feel anything at all.
>
> THERAPIST: Kind of like emotional anesthesia?
>
> FRANK: Right.
>
> THERAPIST: What are the advantages of being numb?
>
> FRANK: Well, you can't get hurt. That's one.
>
> THERAPIST: I see.
>
> FRANK: And you don't feel sad or mad, either.
>
> THERAPIST: I get it. What is the down side?
>
> FRANK: I guess you'd also miss the excitement and good feelings in life. Even though it is like a roller coaster sometimes.
>
> THERAPIST: Yes, I can see how you'd really miss that.

Identifying and Labeling Emotions

The ability to recognize and label a feeling is the first step toward being able to manage it. After all, it is a challenge to effectively manage an emotion you cannot label. We therefore begin emotion regulation by enhancing the teen's ability to accurately identify and label emotions.

The therapist may begin by asking the teen to identify and describe commonly experienced emotions, as well as those that the teen has difficulty tolerating or regulating. How does he or she experience each emotion? The therapist should explore with the teen what he or she notices physiologically, cognitively, and behaviorally. For example:

> THERAPIST: So you were talking about what it feels like when you get angry ...
>
> TEEN: Right. So I feel real hot. My face gets red and my ears start to feel like they are burning. Other people tell me I look red, too.
>
> THERAPIST: OK, and what are you thinking when that is going on for you?
>
> TEEN: Oh, I am usually thinking that the person who ticked me off is going to pay.

The Nature of Emotions

There are three components of emotion regulation that account for individual differences in emotional experience. Emotional responses can be likened to a snowball rolling down a hill:

1. *FAST (threshold and speed of response)*. For some individuals, it does not take much in the way of stress to elicit an emotional response. A mild disappointment for one person might not result in much of an emotional response, but in another person who is more sensitive, a slight nudge can get the snowball rolling. There is very little time between the precipitant and the emotional response—the snowball starts rolling really fast.
2. *BIG (size of the response)*. The intensity of the emotional response is big; emotions are felt and expressed with much intensity, making it difficult to think clearly. And when the emotional snowball gets rolling down the hill, it becomes a BIG snowball.
3. *SLOW (how quickly is the response over?)*. For some individuals, even strong emotions end very quickly. For others, there is a very SLOW return to being calm or relaxed. That is, it takes a long time to roll the snowball back up the hill; it may have done damage as it sped down the hill. So, the teen may now have more distress than he or she had initially (i.e., the emotional experience and subsequent behavior may have made things worse).

The person with emotion dysregulation has a low threshold for an emotional response, the response happens quickly and is intense, and the person is slow to return to a calm baseline.

It is important to help the teen understand that until the snowball is returned to the top of the hill and order is restored, he or she may be more vulnerable to other intense emotions. Subsequently, the teen may respond with intense emotions to the next stressor that comes along. The therapist can prompt the teen for examples of each of these elements of an emotional response.

MADDIE: So, Joe and I had this big fight. I was so mad at him. Just thinking about it right now, I am getting all worked up again.

THERAPIST: OK. And then you came home …

MADDIE: … and my mom started in on me for being late. And I just lost it.

THERAPIST: Right. What did that look like exactly?

MADDIE: Well, I stomped upstairs, and I was yelling and calling her names. Then I slammed my bedroom door so hard behind me that the door broke off one of the hinges.

THERAPIST: I gotcha. It's a little like wading in the surf. If you are still off balance from the wave that came beforehand, it's so much easier for the next wave that comes by to knock you over.

MADDIE: Yup, that's exactly what happened.

Vulnerability to Emotional Dysregulation

Now that the teen understands the elements of an emotionally dysregulated response, the therapist can help the teen identify factors that make those FAST, BIG, and SLOW responses more likely to occur—we refer to these as *vulnerability factors*. The therapist and teen will have already identified some *vulnerability factors* for suicidal behavior via the chain analysis. Common examples of this might be sleep deprivation, substance use, or emotional or physical pain.

The therapist can ask for examples of times the teen was more likely to become cranky or angry because of not taking good care of him- or herself (e.g., "When I don't sleep well, I get more cranky"). The therapist can then invite the teen to consider how he or she might attend to vulnerability factors in order to decrease the likelihood of dysregulation.

Recognizing Emotional Action Urges

All emotions come with action urges that "tell" us to do something—
known as *action urges*. Two vital steps in learning emotion regulation
skills are first to *recognize* common action urges associated with each
emotion, and then to understand that one can learn to *resist* urges.
For example, the action urge associated with fear is often to hide; with
anger, it is to attack; and for sadness, it is to withdraw. The therapist can
use this introduction to then talk with the teen about action urges associated with emotions he or she commonly experiences. The therapist
should highlight that experiencing a strong urge to act in a certain way
does not mean that we have to act on it. Instead, we have choices about
how we act in response to our emotions.

When introducing emotion regulation skills to a depressed and
suicidal teen, the therapist should first identify and reinforce skills the
teen already has in his or her repertoire for regulating negative affect:
"So I know there are already several things you do when you are having
a really hard time—like listening to music or talking to your friends.
What we want to do is try to find some additional tools for you to use
that can come in handy when you are experiencing a lot of emotional
distress." The following are useful techniques for helping teens to tolerate and regulate emotional distress.

THE EMOTIONS THERMOMETER

The emotions thermometer is a visual aid to help the teen understand
that all emotional experience occurs along a continuum. Although individuals may have emotional responses that fall into the FAST, BIG, and
SLOW categories, there usually is some buildup in emotional intensity
prior to reaching the point of loss of control (referred to as the emotional "boiling point"). The thermometer is a tool for visualizing the
range of intensity of emotions. The goal of the emotions thermometer
exercise is to help the teen regulate emotions by learning to "take his or
her emotional temperature" and have steps for "lowering the temperature" prior to reaching the boiling point.

To introduce this exercise to the teen, the therapist can explain
that the intensity of our emotions can be thought of as corresponding
to temperatures that can be charted on a thermometer. The basic skills
for the teen to learn in this exercise are:

1. Taking his or her emotional temperature.
2. Identifying cognitive, behavioral, and emotional correlates of a given temperature.
3. Identifying a "boiling point" or "point of no return" beyond which he or she feels out of control.
4. Developing some simple strategies for reducing emotional temperature prior to reaching the boiling point.

Specific Steps for Teaching the Emotions Thermometer Skill

1. Start by using a blank thermometer (Figure 6.2) and ask the teen to name the way he or she feels when about to lose control. For some it will be "stressed" or "out of control," and for others "frustrated" or "angry." Label one end of the emotions thermometer with this term and the opposite end with "feeling in control" or "relaxed."
2. At each interval, ask the teen to identify physiological, psychological, and behavioral cues that correspond to these markers. Physiological markers might be things like increased heart rate or sweating, psychological cues might be certain thoughts and experiencing action urges, and behavioral cues might be increasing speech volume, clenching fists, or even throwing things.
3. Ask the teen to identify and mark on the thermometer the "boiling point" or "point of no return." Beyond this level, the teen is no longer able to regulate and feels out of control. The physiological, psychological, and behavior markers for this point on the thermometer are then identified.
4. Ask the teen to identify cues that correspond to in-between markers (e.g., 20, 40).
5. Ask the teen to choose a point and accompanying cues that will serve as a signal that he or she needs to "do something" to calm down in order to prevent getting to the identified boiling point or point of no return. This is the point at which he or she is still able to use skills to avoid an outburst or explosion. Label this as the "action point" (there may be more than one "action point").
6. Work with the teen to identify specific steps to take at the action point that will help him or her to control the escalation. These may include behaviors such as taking a walk or listening to music and calming self-talk.

We now describe techniques to use at the "action point."

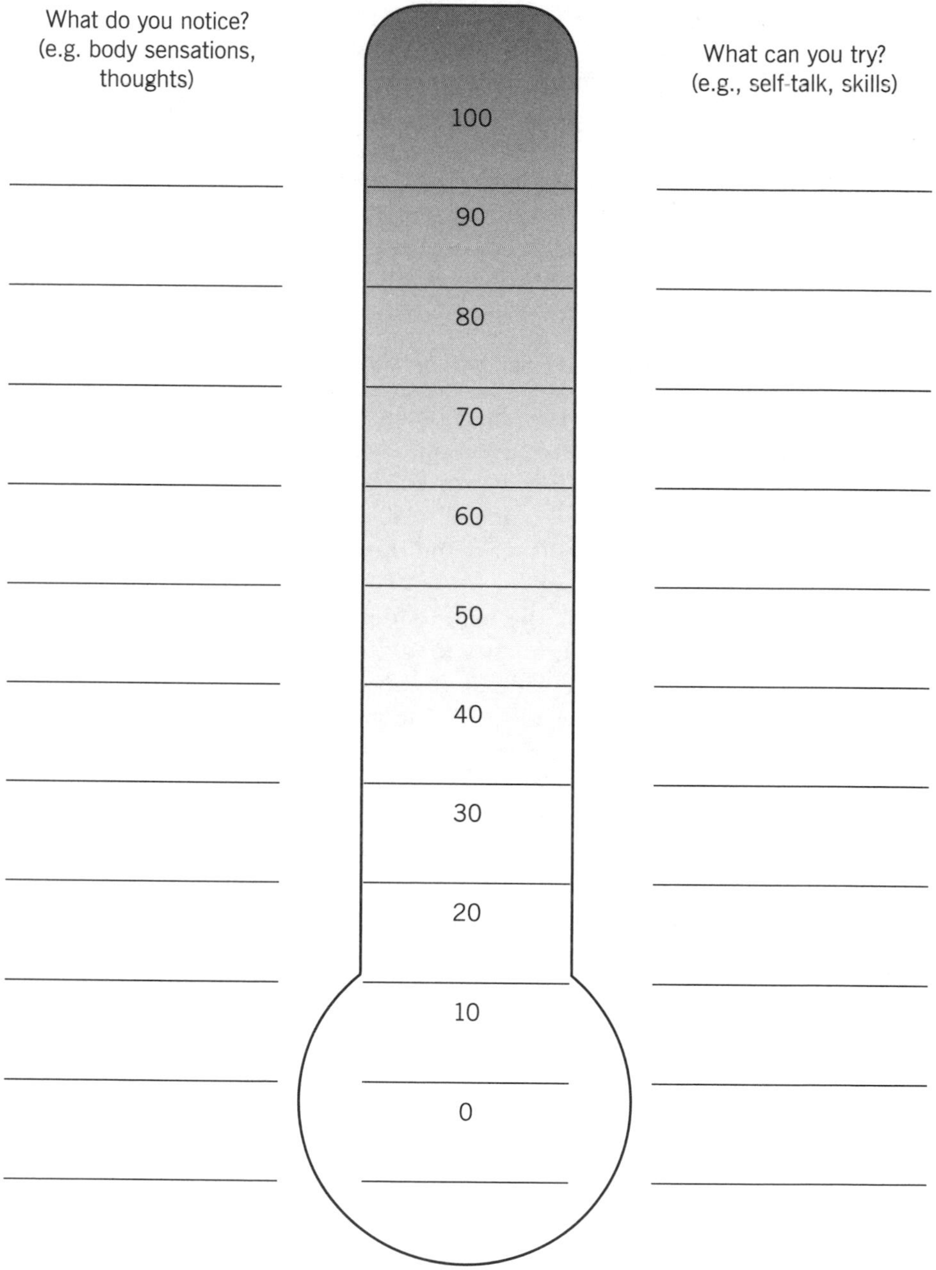

What do you notice?
(e.g. body sensations,
thoughts)

What can you try?
(e.g., self-talk, skills)

100

90

80

70

60

50

40

30

20

10

0

FIGURE 6.2. Emotions thermometer.

DISTRACTION

Distraction can be a powerful technique for psychologically removing oneself temporarily from upsetting thoughts or feelings. The therapist can have the teen identify things he or she already does to distract from upsetting thoughts or feelings. Then the therapist can help identify new behaviors that the teen would be willing to try.

Distraction can be practiced in session by having the teen think about a situation that is sad or upsetting. Next, the therapist can have the teen throw him- or herself into another activity. This could be writing, looking at a magazine, or playing a game. The therapist should ask again how the teen feels, and link the distracting activity to the notion that he or she is no longer thinking about the upsetting situation. The therapist and teen can generate a list of distractions that the teen is willing to try. It is also important for the therapist to make clear to the teen that not every type of distraction will work for every person or for every emotion. Therefore, the teen will need to experiment with various types of distraction in order to determine what will work best for him or her in a given set of circumstances.

SELF-SOOTHING

Another way to distract oneself from upsetting thoughts or feelings is to think about self-soothing through each of the senses. This is a particularly useful exercise for increasing distress tolerance. The therapist should encourage the teen to identify a soothing activity that involves each of the five senses and then practice the activities in session. For example, the therapist can bring in hand lotion (touch), flowers (smell), a piece of hard candy (taste), soft music (sound), and pictures from nature (sight) as examples of sensory self-soothing.

DEEP BREATHING

Deep breathing is a very helpful skill because it is a simple and quick way to relax that can be done anywhere, at any time. The therapist can begin by explaining to the teen that breathing slowly and deeply can have a calming effect. The therapist can model deep breathing for the teen by placing one hand over the stomach; the movement of the hand on the belly as it rises and falls demonstrates the action of breathing. Now the therapist can practice with the teen, as follows: "Breathe in through the nose, filling the lungs completely. Then breathe out through the mouth in a steady and controlled manner." During the practice, the therapist can also suggest that the teen add a cue word or a sentence during deep breathing to enhance the relaxation effects. The word can be said aloud softly or in his or her head. Examples include "relax," "chill," "settle down," "it's OK." As the therapist and teen practice in session, the therapist can offer the teen feedback about his or her breathing to ensure that it is coming from the belly rather than the chest, and that it is slow and controlled.

PROGRESSIVE MUSCLE RELAXATION

Progressive muscle relaxation (PMR) has been widely used to treat anxiety and is therefore particularly beneficial for suicidal and depressed teens with comorbid anxiety. The therapist can start by explaining to the teen that many people tend to tense their muscles when they are stressed or upset, and that this is a normal response to strong emotions. Next, the therapist can explain that relaxation can be tied to the fight-or-flight response: when we are stressed or upset, our bodies react as if we are in danger and get ready for action—even if we don't really need to act. Teens can be prompted to think about how they notice tension in their bodies when they are stressed. Perhaps a teen gets headaches or stomachaches—somatic complaints are common among depressed teens. This skill helps calm the body by focusing on muscle tension. By relaxing our muscles, we can calm down and get our bodies back under control. Here, we present a PMR script. The therapist can go through the script in session with the teen to demonstrate.

> "First settle into a comfortable position. Let all your muscles relax; they should feel loose and heavy. Close your eyes and take three deep, slow breaths. As you breathe in slowly, concentrate on the air as it fills your lungs, and as you breathe out slowly, notice your breath rushing out through your nose and mouth. Breathe in slowly, thinking about the feeling of the air passing in and out of your body. Now, I want you to clench your right fist as tight as you can, and hold it while I count down from 5 ... pay attention to the tight feeling in your fist as I begin to count ... 5 ... 4 ... 3 ... 2 ... 1 ... relax your fist and notice the feeling of soft warmth and relaxation that flows through your fingers into your arm ... pay attention to the feeling of relaxation that fills your arm ... Now clench your left hand into a fist and hold it while I count down from 5 ... pay attention to the

tight feeling in your arm ... 5 ... 4 ... 3 ... 2 ... 1 ... release your fist and notice how the tight feeling leaves your arm and is replaced by the warm, heavy feeling of relaxation. Now hunch your shoulders so they press against your head and neck, and pay attention to the tight feeling this causes as I count down from 5 ... 5 ... 4 ... 3 ... 2 ... 1 ... As you relax your shoulders, pay attention to the warm soothing feeling of relaxation that runs down your head, neck, and shoulders. Now I want you to scrunch up your face like you bit something really sour, like a lemon. Wrinkle up your forehead, and hold it while I count down from 5 ... pay attention to the tightness in your forehead while I count down 5 ... 4 ... 3 ... 2 ... 1 ... relax your forehead now, smoothing out all the wrinkles. Notice how smooth and relaxed your face feels. Now clench your jaws. Bite your teeth together and hold it while I count down ... 5 ... 4 ... 3 ... 2 ... 1 ... now relax. Now I want you to tense up your whole body, from your scrunched-up face to your hunched shoulders, to your tight fists and arms, stiff back and tight stomach, tight legs, and curled-up toes. Make your whole body tense and stiff as a board and hold it while I count down 5 ... 4 ... 3 ... 2 ... 1 ... now let go and relax. Just relax and feel how warm and heavy your whole body feels. Enjoy the relaxing feelings in your body. [Let the teen sit quietly for a minute.] OK, now I would like you to open your eyes and start bringing your body back to normal. Stretch if you need to."

The therapist should inquire about how the exercise felt and explain that it takes some practice to get the hang of, but PMR is a very effective way to manage intense emotion. Like all of the techniques described in this chapter, this technique takes practice. The therapist may consider making an audiotape for the teen that leads him or her through the exercise. In this way, the teen can practice at home. Together, the teen and therapist should agree on a practice schedule. Initially, the teen may consider practicing PMR a few times a week at a set time. The teen can then report back about each practice session and what he or she noticed. The aim is for the teen to become skilled at PMR so that when anxiety or other negative affect arises, these skills can be called to mind and utilized, no matter where he or she is.

PLEASANT IMAGERY

With pleasant imagery, we use our imaginations to calm our bodies by thinking about a relaxing and peaceful scene or place. Different people will find different scenes soothing. The therapist might ask the teen what place he or she finds most relaxing. Get specifics! "Where is it? What time of day is it? What temperature is it? Who are you with? What can you hear? What can you smell? What can you feel?" The therapist should encourage the teen to use all five senses to make the scene as real as possible. The therapist may have the teen write down the relaxing scene, or even draw it if he or she prefers. The teen can practice in session by closing his or her eyes and mentally "going" to the relaxing place. Afterwards, the therapist can ask about how the teen feels, and whether there is a noticeable change in his or her emotional state, heart rate, breathing, and so forth.

EMOTION REGULATION SKILLS WITH THE FAMILY

Often, the emotional intensity in the family of depressed teens can be high, in which case it may be useful to teach emotion regulation techniques not only to the teen individually, but to the parents as well. Therefore, each of the skills described above can be presented to the entire family unit. In addition, there are two emotion regulation strategies that we have found to be particularly helpful in working with parents who experience emotional dysregulation.

Exiting and Waiting

The discussion of the "exit and wait" strategy can be done in session with the teen present or with the parents in a separate session. The idea behind this strategy can be presented to the parents as follows:

> "Whenever you feel your emotions are getting too intense in response to something your teenager said or did, you may find it helpful to exit the situation and wait until both you and your teen are calm enough to resume the discussion."

The therapist should work with the parents to identify their own "action points" and likely interactions that may trigger such a response. The teen and family should discuss this openly; this is a strategy that can be used by all parties. Before exiting the room, the parents should be encouraged to make a brief statement to the teen in which the unacceptable behavior is identified clearly and the teen is informed that the parents are leaving the situation until everyone is calm enough to have a productive discussion.

Staying Short and to the Point

Many parents of depressed teens report that they engage in discussions with their teen during which they find themselves rationalizing (and sometimes arguing) about the same things over and over. One strategy to consider under these circumstances is a general rule of staying short and to the point. Parents can be encouraged to briefly state a specific rule or consequence and then exit the situation instead of lapsing into lectures, criticisms, or rationales. To help parents stay short and to the point, the therapist may help them ensure that rules and consequences are clearly defined in the family. This way, parents can reference these rules, avoid extended explanations to the teen, and avoid becoming dysregulated themselves.

KEY POINTS

- Behavioral activation is helpful for depressed teens who have low energy or have become disengaged.

- Encourage the depressed teen to pursue activities even though he or she may not "feel like" doing things.

- Education about emotions enables the teen to better understand and identify what he or she is feeling.

- Decreasing self-judgments about our emotions can help decrease emotional pain.

- Emotionally dysregulated responses have three main components: BIG, FAST, and SLOW return to baseline.

- Every emotion has an associated action urge.

- The emotion thermometer can be used to help teach distress tolerance and emotion regulation.

CHAPTER 7

Cognitive Restructuring,
Problem Solving,
and Interpersonal Effectiveness

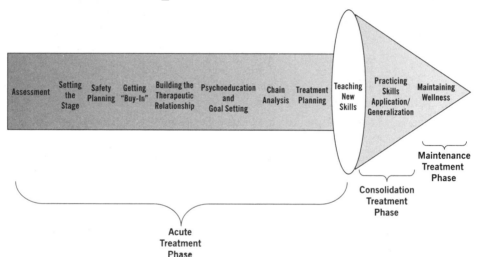

WHAT YOU WILL LEARN IN THIS CHAPTER

- How to help the teen understand that thoughts affect mood and behavior.
- How to help the teen learn to "catch" his or her own cognitive distortions and negative automatic thoughts.
- How to help the teen learn to "rethink" situations to determine if there are alternative ways of interpreting them.
- How to help the teen learn to think in more realistic ways that are more hopeful and positive.
- How to use the chain analysis to explore and challenge key thoughts reported during the past suicidal episode.

- The importance of taking a collaborative approach when determining home-work.
- How to teach and practice the steps for problem solving.
- Important strategies for helping the teen enhance interpersonal skills.

WAYS OF CHANGE

Thoughts, feelings, and actions are interrelated. Intervention with any one of these components can result in change in the other two. Intervention at the level of feelings involves emotion regulation skills, described in Chapter 6. One type of intervention at the level of actions is behavioral activation, also described in more detail in Chapter 6. In this chapter, we focus primarily on intervention at the level of thoughts. There is no clear formula for determining which level of intervention is right for which patient. However, use of the chain analysis to guide treatment planning serves as the foundation. It is also important for the therapist to be flexible enough to recognize when intervention at one level is not working, and to consider the possibility of switching strategies.

COGNITION AND EMOTIONAL DISORDERS

Cognitive therapy is based on the concept that the way we think affects the way we feel, and subsequently the way we behave (though not, of course, always in that order). Early in treatment, it is important to socialize the teen to this basic premise. Depressed teens often show biases in their thinking patterns that tend to reinforce their depression. Suicidal youth show patterns of thinking that reinforce their view that suicide is the only solution to their difficulties. These biases are often referred to as *cognitive distortions*. The process of identifying and challenging these cognitive distortions is a very important component of CBT, and is referred to as *cognitive restructuring*. The depressed teen cannot look for and challenge cognitive distortions unless he or she knows what they are. Therefore, the therapist can first help the teen understand how his or her own thinking is currently affecting mood. It is equally instructive for the teen to learn about patterns of thinking that tend to reinforce depression, as well as those that are helpful in combating depression. Initially in treatment, we do not usually label thoughts as "distorted," but instead help the teen identify "helpful" and "unhelpful" thoughts.

LINKS BETWEEN THINKING, FEELING, AND ACTING

Just talking about the links between thoughts, feelings, and behavior is not likely to result in behavior change. In order to illustrate the interrelationship of thinking, feeling, and behavior, the therapist needs to help the patient to experience this link firsthand. This is consistent with the overall orientation of CBT, termed *collaborative empiricism,*—meaning that the patient and therapist together will evaluate different perspectives on a patient's problems and sift through the evidence in order to find a perspective that is both adaptive and accurate. To illustrate this link, it is best to begin with a concrete example from the patient's recent experience. One effective starting point is to ask the patient for a recent experience that involved an intense emotion, such as sadness or anger. The therapist can then use the teen's example to *differentiate* thoughts, feelings, and behaviors, and then explore the interrelationship among these three facets of experience, as in the following exchange:

THERAPIST: Can you think of a recent time that you experienced an intense emotion?

TEEN: Absolutely. My best friend and I had a huge argument at school today—I am so mad at her.

THERAPIST: I am sorry to hear that … would you like to tell me about what happened?

TEEN: We are always fighting lately—I just think she doesn't care about me. I think she must have a new best friend but she doesn't want to tell me. I am just not going to talk to her again.

THERAPIST: Wow, that sounds really upsetting. How have you been feeling since the fight?

TEEN: I am very sad—but mad too. We have been best friends for over 4 years. We have been through a lot together. I just can't deal with this—I can't even think about talking to her again. It's time for this relationship to end!

THERAPIST: This sounds like something that may be important for us to discuss further. Right now, would it be OK if we used this example to understand thoughts, feelings, and behavior in the here and now?

TEEN: OK.

THERAPIST: What are you feeling about this experience?

TEEN: Mad and sad.

THERAPIST: Both?

TEEN: Mad that my friend is treating me this way, and sad because it isn't the way it used to be.

THERAPIST: You miss the friend you used to have.

TEEN: Right.

THERAPIST: And when that thought goes through your head, how do you feel?

TEEN: Like I said, sad. And also mad, because it doesn't have to be this way.

THERAPIST: And when you feel sad and mad, how does that affect the way you act?

TEEN: I don't want to be around her.

THERAPIST: And what happens then?

TEEN: I miss her more, and feel even more sad and mad about it.

THERAPIST: It goes round and round, doesn't it? Let's recap. You think about missing your old friendship, it makes you feel sad, and you withdraw from her more. Is that right?

CATCHING THE LINK IN REAL TIME

In order to become skilled at identifying thoughts and their relationship to emotions, the therapist should have the teen practice with a couple of other examples to show that this concept can be applied to any situation. The best time and place to build this awareness is during the session. Sudden mood shifts that occur within the session provide an excellent opportunity to illustrate the links between thoughts and feelings. When there is a noticeable shift in mood, the therapist can ask, "What just went through your mind?" or "What thought did you just have?" The thoughts that go along with these affective shifts are sometimes referred to as *hot cognitions*. The therapist can ask the teen to try and notice any shift in mood that occurs between sessions and to keep track of situations and specific thoughts in order to build his or her skills in recognizing unhelpful thoughts. An example of a thought sheet that can be given to the teen for homework is presented in Figure 7.1 (adapted from Beck, 1976, and Beck, 1995).

Once the therapist helps the teen to understand how his or her thoughts are affecting mood and behavior, the therapist can then help

Event	Thought	Emotion and rating (1–10)	Realistic counterthought	Emotion and rating (1–10)

FIGURE 7.1. Thought record.

the teen learn to identify patterns in thinking and behaving that may reinforce depressive feelings. To continue with the example of our patient who is experiencing disappointment with a close friend:

THERAPIST: What are you thinking about your friendship right now?

TEEN: It's hopeless. There is nothing to be done, and my friendship with her is over.

THERAPIST: And then you feel sad?

TEEN: Right.

THERAPIST: So let's just say for the moment that the friendship is not totally hopeless and that maybe there could be some other explanations for the recent conflict. If that was the case, would you feel differently?

TEEN: Sure, but she's really being mean.

THERAPIST: Clearly, this is a very upsetting situation. It sounds like she has been someone very important to you. You have been best friends for a long time. Have you two had disagreements in the past?

TEEN: Yeah, but not this bad.

THERAPIST: How did you work it out in the past?

TEEN: Well, I'm not sure—it just seemed to work out somehow.

THERAPIST: Do you think there could be any other explanations for why she is acting the way she has been?

TEEN: I don't know. I don't think so.

THERAPIST: Well, I don't know either, but maybe we could take a look together and see if we can identify any other ways to think about this situation. Often our first thoughts—we call these *automatic thoughts*—seem accurate, especially when our emotions are strong. However, sometimes if we evaluate our conclusions, we may find other explanations, or at least other ways to think about the situation, that make it a little less painful.

At this point in treatment, we find it very important to emphasize that the process of identifying and evaluating thinking patterns is not intended to simply mean "think positively." Nor is the therapist trying to tell the patient *what* to think. Instead, the therapist is trying to teach the teen that there are alternative ways to think about a given situation—in other words, to help the teen "rethink" the situation and consider all possible explanations. Then it is up to the teen, with the guidance of the therapist, to decide which of these alternatives best fits the facts. The process of considering different explanations for a given situation—such as a big change in a relationship with a friend—can itself reduce the intensity of emotion.

> TEEN: So maybe if I thought about it differently, I might feel better?
>
> THERAPIST: Well, how do you think that would work?
>
> TEEN: I'm not sure. I mean, it would make me feel a little like some kind of a robot or something, like I was not entitled to have my feelings.
>
> THERAPIST: The idea of being like a robot is a great example—could you go further with that?
>
> TEEN: A robot is programmed to do things, and it just does them without any other options.
>
> THERAPIST: As compared to …
>
> TEEN: People have a choice. We can think what we want and feel what we want.
>
> THERAPIST: You are so right. Our goal is for you to be able to be free to have a full range of thoughts and feelings. But if the negative thoughts predominate, then it seems like you are actually being controlled by your thoughts, rather than vice versa. If you look at the situation and come to the conclusion that things really are hopeless—well, sometimes they are and it is good to know that. But maybe you don't want to jump to that conclusion and lose a friend that you have known most of your life if perhaps the negative thought is not entirely accurate.
>
> TEEN: I guess I see what you are saying.

Once teens begin to see the connections between how they think, feel, and behave, the therapist can get more precise about identifying and exploring specific thinking patterns that are predominant—in particular, those potentially related to the problems that brought the patient into therapy in the first place. The rationale is that certain patterns of thinking about oneself, the future, and the world can lead a person to feel more depressed. However, it is critical to emphasize the fact that, although challenging at times, these patterns can be modified in order to help the person feel better. Providing this rationale is important, so that the patient can begin to understand that there can be a powerful payoff to identifying and challenging patterns of thinking that reinforce depression or suicidal ideation and behavior. One analogy that we have used with our patients involves sledding. The therapist can illustrate a common sledding experience—once a downhill sledding pathway has been created in the snow, sledders tend to stay in that same pathway every time they go down the hill on the sled. We then make the link between patterns of thinking and the sledding path. That is, our thinking tends to go down a similar pathway time after time if we are not actively steering in a different direction. Often when people are depressed, their thinking patterns can get stuck in a pathway that maintains their depressed mood. By becoming aware of this tendency, we can learn to steer out of a pathway that is likely to lead to depression.

COGNITIVE DISTORTIONS

At this point, the therapist has helped the teen understand the concept of helpful and unhelpful thinking patterns and their connection to mood. Now, he or she can help the teen to identify some common thinking patterns that go along with depression. The therapist should reinforce the idea that there is almost always more than one way to look at things. Many people get stuck in unhelpful thinking pathways when they only think in one way and forget about or do not take notice of other ways of thinking about things. For example, an individual may miss positive information, fail to notice good things that are happening, or think about things as absolutely good and absolutely bad. These are examples of cognitive distortions. *Cognitive distortions* are systematic errors in reasoning or logic that often become exaggerated during times of psychological distress. For this reason, we often use emotion regulation techniques in addition to cognitive techniques to make it easier for patients to process and let go of their cognitive distortions. Cognitive distortions cause people to process their experiences in a way that causes and/or maintains a depressed mood. To illustrate, a person might be in a supermarket checkout line, and the cashier does not smile at him. A helpful thought, free of distortion, may be "The cashier is grumpy. She must be really busy," whereas a depressed person might think, "She doesn't like me."

Sometimes a thought may appear to be a distortion but in fact is consistent with reality. Some patients are either so irritable or have such poor social skills that, indeed, very few people like them. A patient with a learning disability may indeed feel like a failure because he or she cannot keep up with a typical academic load. A patient with a parent who is a drug addict and homeless may be in a situation that is very unlikely to change. Since the approach to every possible cognitive distortion is to test that thought against the evidence, the therapist and patient need to be open to the possibility that the patient's perception is not a distortion. If that is the case, the therapeutic approach becomes more about helping the patient cope with a particular set of challenges, as compared to testing, challenging, and modifying dysfunctional patterns of thinking.

AUTOMATIC THOUGHTS, ASSUMPTIONS, AND CORE BELIEFS

Practically speaking, how can the therapist teach the patient to catch cognitive distortions before they cascade into changes in mood and behavior? Patients need to be taught to recognize what are termed *automatic thoughts*. Automatic thoughts are reflexive and uncensored, and occur constantly in response to both internal and external triggers. Automatic thoughts are not necessarily dysfunctional, but if a patient is prone to cognitive distortions, then his or her automatic thoughts will reflect those distortions. Furthermore, because automatic thoughts occur so quickly and reflexively, they often go unchallenged, as if they represent the truth. If an automatic thought reflects a depressive bias, then that thought, unmonitored, can set into motion a pattern of additional thoughts, feelings, and actions based on biased assumptions. Since these automatic thoughts tend to occur outside of a patient's awareness, one of the first key interventions for the therapist using a CBT model is to teach the patient to recognize automatic thoughts so that it will be possible to monitor and challenge distorted ones before they take on a life of their own. Here is an example of a therapist teaching a patient to recognize automatic thoughts.

> THERAPIST: I am sorry to hear that you almost made a suicide attempt. Could we review what was going on that led up to that?
>
> TEEN: I called my girlfriend to hang out, and she told me she didn't want to date me anymore.
>
> THERAPIST: Just like that?
>
> TEEN: She said I was too clingy and demanding, and she wanted out.
>
> THERAPIST: That must have hurt.

TEEN: Really. I thought, I really need her to be my girlfriend, and if she's not, then I might as well kill myself.

THERAPIST: Wait, you lost me. How did you get from needing this girl to be your girlfriend to killing yourself?

TEEN: Oh, I thought, "Without her, I'm nothing."

THERAPIST: And because you're nothing, you should die.

TEEN: Right.

THERAPIST: Let's take a snapshot of your brain right there. This thought—"Without her, I'm nothing"—just popped into your head?

TEEN: Yeah.

THERAPIST: And, at the time, how sure were you that this was true?

TEEN: 90%.

THERAPIST: And now?

TEEN: 30%.

THERAPIST: Still a lot, but also a lot less. What changed?

TEEN: I'm calmer, and I realized there is more to life than just having her as my girlfriend.

THERAPIST: That thought you had, "Without her, I'm nothing"—we call that an *automatic thought*. When you have one of those, if it represents depressive thinking, then you tend to buy into it without thinking about it. Then you feel worse, and might even do something drastic.

TEEN: But they happen so fast—and it seemed so true.

THERAPIST: So we need to find ways of catching them and recognizing them so that they don't cause you such suffering.

Automatic thoughts are the end product of two deeper psychological phenomena: core beliefs and assumptions. We all have core beliefs—both functional and dysfunctional. By definition, a *core belief* is thought by the patient to be true, and will cause that patient to take action and interpret events in accordance with that belief, regardless of external facts. Often, a core belief has a basis in truth based on previous experiences, and may have even been adaptive. However, if circumstances shift, and the belief does not, then that core belief may become maladaptive. For example, an adult who was abused as a child may have core beliefs like "The world is a dangerous place" and "People are not to be trusted." If the person is in an environment where he or she might be hit at any time, then these are adaptive assumptions. In fact, having a naïve and trusting attitude under such circumstances could be life threatening. However, when that child grows up and gets a job and has to work as part of a team, being suspicious and quick to conclude that others are hostile can be maladaptive. Core beliefs are about the self, the world, and the future. A core belief about the self would be in the form of an "I am" statement, such as "I am unlovable." A belief about the world would be like the example described above, "People are not to be trusted." A core belief about the future would be "The future is hopeless."

Core beliefs then give rise to a phenomenon that serves as an intermediary between beliefs and automatic thoughts—*assumptions*. Assumptions are if/then statements that relate to the self, the world, or the future. For example, "If I don't have a girlfriend, then nobody really cares about me."

The interrelationship between thoughts, assumptions, and core beliefs, as illustrated in Figure 7.2, is like a tree. The automatic thoughts are the end products, or leaves, the most accessible part. The assumptions are like branches, and the core beliefs like the trunk and roots. Core beliefs give rise to assumptions that then give rise to automatic thoughts. To return to the example of the boy who almost made a suicide attempt because he was rejected by his girlfriend: his automatic thought was "Without her [as my girlfriend], I'm nothing." This automatic thought was one about himself—being "nothing" or "worthless." His assumption turned out to be "Unless someone loves me, I am worthless." His core belief about himself was that he was "worthless."

The teen will share his or her experience of, and most easily report on, his or her automatic thoughts. In our analogy, automatic thoughts are the leaves because they are immediately evident and readily accessible. Let's return to the patient who was really upset about relationship difficulties with her close friend.

THERAPIST: So when your friend snubs you, what are you thinking?

TEEN: Friendships never work out for me.

THERAPIST: Really, I thought you had been friends for years.

TEEN: Yeah, but in the end, look what happened.

THERAPIST: Would you say this says something about you, or about other people?

TEEN: It says that other people are no good, and will always turn on you.

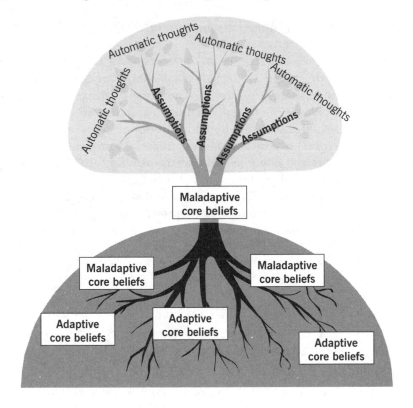

FIGURE 7.2. The CBT tree.

THERAPIST: And if you do trust someone?

TEEN: Then they will eventually hurt you.

The automatic thought this girl is describing is "Relationships never work for me." The assumption is "If you trust people, you'll get hurt." The core belief is "People can't be trusted." In the beginning stages of therapy, the therapist is listening for automatic thoughts. The therapist then leads the teen through three steps: identifying, exploring, and modifying the automatic thoughts (leaves). We want to stress that a treatment focused solely on this work with automatic thoughts will, most often, lead to symptom relief. However, for many youth, sustained relief and protection from relapse requires delving deeper to address assumptions and core beliefs—the branches and trunk and roots of the tree. In relatively brief treatment, it is most often not possible to modify core beliefs. However, the patient can become aware of them and be ready to counter the assumptions and automatic thoughts produced by these beliefs.

Core beliefs serve as the "trunk and roots of the tree" because they are underlying the automatic thoughts, less readily accessible, and serve to *feed* the tree branches and leaves. The same three steps utilized to work with automatic thoughts—identify, explore, and modify—are also applied to addressing core beliefs. It is important to share with the teen that everyone has core beliefs, both adaptive and maladaptive. For example, a depressed boy who feels worthless might still have a belief that his parents care about him and want what is best for him. The ability to access positive and adaptive beliefs and skills is compromised by the experience of depressed mood. Therefore, when a patient becomes depressed, the unhelpful or maladaptive beliefs tend to predominate, even though the adaptive beliefs are still extant. An exploration of reasons for living as part of the assessment can give clues as to adaptive beliefs.

> THERAPIST: You found yourself thinking a lot about suicide this week?
>
> TEEN: I felt really down.
>
> THERAPIST: But you did not act on these thoughts. Why?
>
> TEEN: I know it sounds crazy, as difficult as things might be now, but I think, if I can get through this, then I can do something with my life. In fact, I think I would be a really good psychologist. Kids could come to me for help.
>
> THERAPIST: We certainly can use more good psychologists. It's good to hear that this is something that keeps you going.

Assumptions are like the "branches of the tree" in that they serve as the link between automatic thoughts ("leaves") and core beliefs ("trunk and roots"). Ironically, assumptions serve to protect us from confronting our unhelpful core beliefs. For example, a person whose core belief is "I am inadequate" may be protected against feelings of inadequacy by the assumption "If I am perfect at everything I do, then I am OK." As long as the patient keeps doing everything perfectly, or close to it, then the feelings of inadequacy are held at bay. The core beliefs emerge when the person can no longer fulfill the terms of the implicit contract of the assumption.

The tree analogy can be a helpful tool for illustrating the nature of the CBT model. Because of the abstract nature of thoughts and their relationship to core beliefs, drawing the tree can help the teen understand how core beliefs and assumptions may be playing a role in his or her depression.

The key to CBT is catching cognitive distortions and unhelpful automatic thoughts, challenging them, and considering more realistic ways of looking at the world that are more hopeful and less likely to reinforce depression. We do not usually teach or give the teen a list of the common cognitive distortions. Rather, we tend to point out the specific patterns of unhelpful thinking that are prominent for each individual. For therapists, we provide some specific examples of common types of cognitive distortions below:

- *Selective abstraction.* A 14-year-old girl comes home with a graded test with the following comments: "Excellent! Really creative—need to be a little more careful about spelling and grammar." She concludes that the teacher thought the composition was "no good." This would be an example of selective abstraction, in which the individual selectively attends to the negative aspects of a situation and ignores the positive. This makes it very difficult for the individual to feel good about herself.

- *All-or-nothing thinking (or black-and-white thinking).* A ninth-grade boy tries out for the basketball team. Freshmen almost never make the varsity team, but he is selected. However, he is not selected to start for the first game. He decides to quit, thinking, "If I am not a starter, there is no sense in playing." This is an example of all-or-nothing thinking. This student is setting unattainably high expectations for himself and his coach, and depriving himself of the enjoyment of participating and improving.

- *Overgeneralization.* A 17-year-old girl who has usually been a very good student fails an exam. As a consequence, she concludes that she is unlikely to be successful in college. This would be an example of overgeneralization, or drawing sweeping conclusions from an isolated incident.

- *Hopelessness.* A 16-year-old boy wants to go to the prom, and is told by a friend that a particular girl likes him and would like to be asked. He does not call her, thinking, "No one would go out with me anyway." This is an example of hopelessness, a pessimistic view of the future that we have previously described as a risk factor for suicidal behavior. This way of thinking is clearly coloring his view of his chances that she would say yes to him. This thought leads him not to call the girl, and not to go to the prom, thereby confirming his thought that "No one likes me."

SUICIDAL THINKING

Negative automatic thoughts that lead to episodes of suicidality are particularly important to identify. This can be done by revisiting the chain analysis, with an emphasis on identifying key thoughts in the chain to suicidal behavior. During suicidal crises, the teen's thoughts may be related to hopelessness, worthlessness, and powerlessness. Two of the most common motivations for attempting suicide are to die and to escape a painful feeling. Patients who want to die may think, "My family would be better off without me" or "Nothing will ever get better." Patients who want to escape a painful feeling may think, "I can't stand the pain." These cognitive distortions related to suicidal behavior are reflected in the following case examples:

> THERAPIST: You said at the time you made your attempt that you really wanted to die.
>
> TEEN: I still feel that way.
>
> THERAPIST: On a scale of 1–10, if 10 is that you really want to die and 1 is that you don't, where are you at today?
>
> TEEN: 8.
>
> THERAPIST: Why not a 10?
>
> TEEN: I don't know. I guess I was surprised at how concerned my family was. I was thinking that they would be better off without me, but for whatever reason, they seem to think differently.
>
> THERAPIST: So you think there is a slight possibility that they would not think they would be better off without you.
>
> TEEN: Maybe more than that. But I still feel that way.
>
> THERAPIST: Feelings don't make something true—but it makes them feel true!

This second example is about cognitive distortions related to "not being able to stand the pain."

> THERAPIST: You made a really scary suicide attempt.
>
> TEEN: Yeah.
>
> THERAPIST: What was driving you to take such a big step?
>
> TEEN: The emotional pain I was feeling—I just could not stand it.
>
> THERAPIST: You could not stand it ... what did you think would happen if you just kept feeling it?

TEEN: I don't know. But it was worse than physical pain. It just really hurt.

THERAPIST: On a scale of 1–10, if 10 is the worst, how bad was it?

TEEN: 11.

THERAPIST: Yikes, that's terrible. And now?

TEEN: 7.

THERAPIST: So the pain goes up and down?

TEEN: Yeah.

THERAPIST: So having an 11 one day doesn't mean you won't have a 7 a week later.

TEEN: True, but when you have an 11, you are not taking the long view.

THERAPIST: So what is the most pain that you think you could stand?

TEEN: Probably an 8.5 or 9.

THERAPIST: So if we could get your pain down to there, at least for a while, you think you could be safe?

TEEN: Yeah.

THERAPIST: I have another question: The emotional pain you were experiencing—do you think there is anything you, or the two of us, could do to change it?

TEEN: Maybe.

Another issue implicit in the decision to attempt suicide is the thought "There are no other possible solutions." We will discuss how to help suicidal patients improve their ability to generate other alternatives, but first, patients have to believe that there *could* be other solutions.

COGNITIVE RESTRUCTURING

Recognition that one is having cognitive distortions is not enough to result in mood and behavior change. The patient needs to be equipped with the tools to challenge cognitive distortions and counter with other thoughts that are more functional and accurate. This technique is referred to as *cognitive restructuring*, and is at the heart of all forms of CBT. Once the teen is able to see the relationship among thoughts, feelings, and behaviors, and to identify cognitive distortions, the therapist can teach the teen techniques to counter these distortions. The therapist can begin by asking a series of questions designed to help the patient examine alternative perspectives that are more consistent with the available facts and might not lead to such intense distressing emotions. After the teen has been taught some techniques for cognitive restructuring, the teen and therapist can plan experiments in which the teen uses a thought record to identify a cognitive distortion, considers the evidence for and against that automatic thought, and develops a counterthought.

Conversely, a negative thought is not necessarily a cognitive distortion. Our patients often face challenges that are very distressing, and also completely out of their control. The therapist should review with the patient some differences between a distortion and a problem beyond the patient's control. In such cases, the patient can still influence his or her response to the problem, even if he or she is not in a position to solve the problem. For example, a patient may have a parent who is depressed but refuses to get treatment. The patient cannot make the parent better, and the perception that the parent does not act in a loving and supportive manner is based in reality. However, the patient still has a choice about how to cope with the situation.

The therapist can help the teen to discover that often there are alternative ways to look at upsetting situations that may help the teen lessen his or her distress. This realization—that it is possible to change one's thinking patterns—can be a very empowering message for our patients. The therapist should not lose an opportunity to determine whether, after this realization, the patient feels more hopeful about improvement.

Ways to Help Teens Challenge Automatic Thoughts

We have found a variety of techniques to be effective for helping teens challenge, and ultimately modify, their automatic thoughts:

Reviewing the Pros and Cons

For some teens, it may be helpful to start by reviewing the advantages and disadvantages of thinking a certain way. The therapist can help a teen see that there are advantages and disadvantages of holding on to a certain thought or position: "How does that way of thinking work for you?" "Are there any other ways to think about it that might not be as painful for you?" In this way, the therapist can encourage the teen to consider that the automatic thought may not necessarily be true, and that he or she can choose to embrace or dismiss it.

> TEEN: Anyway, I am overwhelmed with schoolwork.
>
> THERAPIST: Did you go to the counselor like we talked about to reduce your courseload?
>
> TEEN: No.
>
> THERAPIST: Oh. Why is that?
>
> TEEN: I really need to keep at the top of my class.
>
> THERAPIST: At the cost of your health?
>
> TEEN: Look, the only way I am worthwhile is if I am doing really well.
>
> THERAPIST: So in order to be worthwhile, you have to be really doing outstanding work.
>
> TEEN: Right.
>
> THERAPIST: Any advantage to holding that perspective?
>
> TEEN: Sure. As long as I keep performing, I feel OK about myself.
>
> THERAPIST: OK, that's important. What's the down side?
>
> TEEN: I don't think I can keep up.
>
> THERAPIST: So, either you have to get by on no sleep, or decide that maybe doing a little less is OK somehow?
>
> TEEN: I am not there yet.
>
> THERAPIST: So, right now, the advantages outweigh the disadvantages?
>
> TEEN: Seems like it.
>
> THERAPIST: OK, so we might want to revisit this, but I'll leave that up to you.

Socratic Questioning

Socratic questioning invites the patient to consider the evidence for a particular thought from a variety of perspectives. The therapist asks questions that will stimulate curiosity within the patient. The questions are open-ended in nature to encourage the patient to sift through the evidence and draw a conclusion. Together, the therapist and patient are trying to discover to what extent a particular thought is valid. Here are a few examples:

- "Are there any other ways to look at the situation?"
- "Is that the only way someone could look at that situation?"
- "How else might someone see that situation?"
- "Could it be that the thought could be partially true?"
- "What evidence do we have that would support the thought? If we were going in front of a judge in a court of law, do you think we could prove it to the judge?"
- "If other people took a look at that thought, what do you think they would say about it?"

Role Play

The therapist and teen can use role play to come up with alternative ways to think through a troubling situation. The therapist can play the role of the teen (this can always be a time to have a laugh at the therapist) and the therapist can model self-questioning. The therapist also can model how to think of alternative explanations or thoughts. The therapist may choose to model in a way that shows the teen how hard it can be to come up with alternative thoughts; this is often much more effective than if the therapist comes up with a quick, unrealistic response. The teen can then return to his or her role and practice what the therapist has modeled. The therapist and teen can make modifications to the plan based on the role play.

THERAPIST: So I'll be you. You be me. OK?

TEEN: Yeah, OK.

THERAPIST: So I was getting ready to go out with some friends, and I thought, "I am not going to have fun anyway."

TEEN: So what did you do?

THERAPIST: Stayed home.

TEEN: When you had the thought, "I am not going to have fun anyway," was there any other way to think about that?

THERAPIST: Well, my friends might be boring, but it has to be better than staying home alone.

TEEN: How could you test that out?

THERAPIST: Next time, say yes and compare.

Recording Alternative Thoughts

The overall goal of any of the techniques described above is to help the teen learn ways to generate alternative thoughts to distressing automatic thoughts. The teen and therapist can write the alternative thoughts on paper, cards, or a whiteboard. The therapist should focus on guiding the teen to think of realistic, less harsh (but not necessarily positive) counter-thoughts that will help the teen combat distressing automatic thoughts. Often the list can be helpful for teens to keep, especially in the early phases of treatment when they may not be as skilled at independently coming up with counterthoughts. In our experience, the most effective strategy for recording alternative thoughts is on index cards (sometimes called *coping cards*; see Beck, 1995), that can be taken home. On the card, we have the patient prepare a list of his or her most common automatic thoughts with some helpful responses (see Figure 7.3).

Some patients believe that "if I think it, it means it's true." They have difficulty distinguishing a thought from a fact. In some instances, this can be due to a strongly ingrained set of beliefs and assumptions. Such patients may be encouraged to consider a thought experiment—to consider the ramifications if the thought were not true. Such patients

THOUGHT	QUESTION	COUNTERTHOUGHT
No one will ever go out with me	Have you asked EVERYONE yet?	Some people might say no, but there are a lot of people I haven't asked.
I'm doomed to be a failure.	Have you really failed at EVERYTHING?	Everyone has setbacks.
I will never be able to recover from this depression.	Has this treatment helped other people with depression?	Lots of people with similar problems have gotten better.
People are no good.	It is possible that there are some good people, but you haven't met them yet?	I can be cautious about people without rejecting them before getting to know them.
Since people are going to laugh at me, I might as well skip this party.	What is the worst that could happen?	Once in a while some people might laugh at me, but would they really be people I should care about?

FIGURE 7.3. Example of coping card.

also may be more amenable to considering advantages and disadvantages, as compared to directly challenging thoughts, assumptions, and beliefs. Or a therapist can ask such a patient, "Given that you believe that this is true, how can we best help you cope with that belief?"

Some patients have a great deal of difficulty with perspective taking. It can also be difficult for teens to see that two people can experience the exact same situation but interpret it quite differently. This may be particularly relevant when a patient is experiencing interpersonal difficulties but is having trouble seeing the perspective of the other party. Role play can help to illustrate this.

Patients can sometimes experience difficulty in labeling and describing emotional and cognitive experiences. Recall may be impaired if the experience itself took place under great duress. Recall can be heightened by inviting the patient to remember as much as possible about the events of the day—the weather, the room, what the patient was wearing. Patients may also have difficulty teasing out different emotions they may have had when they experienced more than one at the same time. The patient may experience more than one strong emotion at once: anger and depression, or anxiety and sadness. The therapist should avoid premature closure when getting the patient to describe his or her experience and be open to the likely possibility that the patient is experiencing more than one emotion at a time.

Homework

The patient can practice taking different perspectives in the office, but it can also be beneficial for him or her to practice taking perspective and generating counterthoughts when at home or at school. Experiments—either behavioral, emotional, or cognitive—in which the teen is asked to notice something or try practicing a new skill are often referred to as *homework*. The therapist and teen can use homework as a way to help the teen notice and challenge automatic thoughts as well as solidify skills and strategies reviewed during sessions. At least initially, many depressed teens in therapy are not overjoyed at the idea of doing therapy homework. Instead of using the term *homework*, we sometimes use alternative terms such as *experiment, collecting data,* or *practice.* Like all other aspects of treatment, homework assignments should be developed collaboratively, and the teen and therapist should brainstorm about possible barriers that might interfere with successful completion. Toward the end of the session, the therapist can ask the teen to summarize the session and collaboratively determine meaningful homework. The therapist should always ask about homework in the following session and be open to feedback if the assignment might need to be restructured.

PROBLEM SOLVING

Effective problem solving has several components: (1) assessment and formulation of the problem; (2) generation of alternative solutions; (3) choosing one solution; (4) implementing that solution; and (5) evaluating how well that solution addressed the problem. Problem solving has been shown to be an important component of CBT, and effective as a stand-alone intervention for depression and for suicidal behavior in adults. Effective problem solving is particularly relevant for suicidal adolescents, who have difficulty generating alternative solutions to suicide in stressful situations. Part of the key to effective problem solving is emotion regulation—that is, helping the patient to identify cues that indicate that he or she is at risk of losing emotional control, and coming up with strategies for managing strong emotions when they arise (see Chapter 6). It is therefore important to identify what emotions could get in the way of effective problem solving and to have a plan for coping with them.

The ability to actively solve problems is an essential skill for all teens. It is especially important for youth who may be exposed to a higher than expected amount of stress and to those with psychiatric or medical chronic illness, in order to optimize their coping with difficulties associated with these disorders. Before implementing training in problem solving, it is important to assess the teen's attitudes and motivation toward learning problem solving. If a teen believes that everything is hopeless, then learning problem solving skills does not make sense, since the teen feels helpless to act on his or her environment. Also, depressed and suicidal teens may come from families with high levels of socioeconomic and psychiatric stress. The patient may justifiably ask why he or she has to try to solve a seemingly overwhelming list of problems. While this feeling is valid, it is also true that even if they did not cause their problems, they nonetheless are left to solve them. It can also be helpful for teens to realize that *some* problems are simply a normal part of life. By becoming skillful at solving problems, the teen will feel more empowered to handle life's challenges—fair and unfair. Furthermore, one of the skills of problem solving is being able to identify the difference between problems that may need to be accepted and those that can actively be solved.

During therapy sessions, the therapist should first introduce the five problem-solving steps to the patient:

1. *Identify the problem:* Be very specific and concretely identify the problem.
2. *Brainstorm all possible options:* Guide the teen to identify as many solutions as possible, without evaluating the solutions. This is a time the therapist can add some ideas, including some that may even be unrealistic or humorous, illustrating the point of brainstorming *every* possible option.
3. *Evaluate pros and cons of all options:* After a complete list has been created, then start to evaluate each. The therapist should work collaboratively with the teen to evaluate the pros and cons of each one, crossing off the ones that seem unlikely choices. Narrow the list to a couple of "finalists."
4. *Decide on one solution and explore potential roadblocks:* Help the teen decide which would be the best solution, given the pros and cons. It is important to point out that any one solution may not be ideal, but can always be modified later as needed. Also decide on what would be the expected outcome of a given solution, so that the efficacy of that solution can be evaluated.
5. *Implement and evaluate:* The therapist should role-play with the teen the steps for putting the plan into action. Evaluate how the role play went and make modifications to the plan as needed. Ask again about any potential roadblocks for implementing the plan. The therapist should also remember to ask about how it went at the next session.

Generalization of Problem-Solving Skills

Once the teen is familiar with the problem-solving steps, he or she should be invited to identify some possible opportunities for trying out these skills. The therapist can help the teen identify and prioritize problems during the session, and then help the teen to pick an experiment to try these skills out. The practice situation should be one in which the patient is likely to experience success. Practice is important because problem solving is always more challenging in real life than during a therapy session. Therefore, using the skill outside of session is an important way to "test out" the acquired skill. Based on the content of the teen's agenda items in session, the therapist can get an idea of how effective the teen has become at problem solving.

Suicidality and Problem Solving

Problem-solving strategies are especially important in the treatment of suicidal teens. First, teens often engage in suicidal behavior because they conclude there are no other options. This may be attributed in part to hopelessness. Also, many adolescent suicide attempters are prone to emotion dysregulation and to impulsive decision making. These two conditions are inconsistent with rational, deliberate problem solving and the ability to generate viable alternatives. Throughout treatment, the therapist can work with the teen to determine the connection between life stressors, depressive symptoms, and suicidality. The therapist and teen can refer back to the initial chain analysis, as well as subsequent chains, to tailor the problem-solving strategies to reduce future suicidal episodes.

For example, if the teen was trying to express anger at his or her parents during a suicidal crisis, finding other means of expressing anger toward parents and/or managing anger will be important to address in treatment. In this situation, problem solving represents a bridge between analyzing the problem and accessing the appropriate requisite skills.

For some suicidal teens, hopelessness may interfere with the ability to learn effective strategies for problem solving. Hopelessness can be targeted directly. Another way to address hopelessness is by helping the teen experience a successful attempt at solving a problem. It can often be helpful to begin by trying to solve a relatively easy problem in session.

Some suicidal teens are also impulsive. The impulsivity has to be slowed down in order for the teen to become an effective problem solver. A patient might carry a coping card that reminds him or her to focus and not to act impulsively, and then lists the five problem-solving steps. The therapist and teen can determine when the impulsive urges tend to occur and work on strategies for riding out such urges. By helping the teen realize that the urges are not constant and will pass with time, the teen can gain confidence with regard to his or her ability to cope with future urges and ward off impulsive acts. The teen may find using skills for regulating emotions to be very helpful for getting through an urge (see Chapter 6). Ultimately, these strategies will help buy time to get through any impulsive urge the teen may experience. Once the teen has passed through the urge, he or she will be more capable of utilizing problem-solving skills. The following is a case example of a 15-year-old boy who seemed to be doing well in CBT but impulsively made a suicide attempt:

THERAPIST: I was really surprised to hear from the emergency room that you had made a suicide attempt.

TEEN: Yeah, I was kinda surprised I did it.

THERAPIST: Really? How were you taken by surprise?

TEEN: I got into a shouting match with my dad, who told me for the millionth time that I will never amount to anything. I just saw red, I was so mad, and took a bunch of my Prozac.

THERAPIST: We had done some serious work on problem solving and generating alternatives. Were you able to use that here?

TEEN: No way! I was just too mad.

THERAPIST: So you are able to remember your problem-solving steps when you are calm, but when you really needed them, you were too upset?

TEEN: Uh-huh.

THERAPIST: Oh, of course I see. It sounds like we can work together on ways to maintain emotional balance so that you can be a more effective problem solver. Can we give that a try now?

ENHANCING INTERPERSONAL SKILLS

The development of interpersonal skills is a critical developmental task for adolescents. It is always helpful to refer back to the initial chain analysis to help the teen see the relevance of enhancing interpersonal skills for both mood and suicidal behavior. Generally, there are several reasons why a focus on interpersonal skills is important for the treatment of depressed and suicidal adolescents. Interpersonal conflicts are often cited as strong contributors to depression, and are precipitants for suicidal behavior. The motivations for adolescent suicide attempts often include interpersonal motivations. Furthermore, the perception of some depressed teens that they are unlikable may reflect a lack of interpersonal effectiveness. Since strong and meaningful social bonds are among the most important protective factors against future depression and suicidal behavior, our patients should be equipped with the ability to forge such bonds. These will be very important for the long-term well-being of our patients. Additionally, enhancing interpersonal skills can be helpful for improving mood and self-confidence.

The most common motivations for adolescent suicide attempts include expressing a feeling, getting someone to pay attention, or otherwise influencing someone's behavior. In all of these motivations, there is a lack of direct communication. A chain analysis can reveal this.

Direct Communication

The therapist has identified that a patient has difficulty directly expressing his or her needs and feelings. The therapist can explain the basics of effective communication, highlighting the following points:

- Make "I" statements, rather than "you" statements.
- Introduce your request before you make it.
- Ask or tell in a calm manner, at a time when the other person is not preoccupied or upset.
- Keep your communication simple. Don't ask for too much at once.
- Reflect back to the other party what you think you heard before giving a response.
- Don't make statements that are generalizations, like "You *always* do this."
- Pay attention to your body language and that of the person to whom you are speaking. Look directly at the person while you are talking.

The following is a case example of a patient who was angry with her parents for putting so much pressure on her academically. She felt as if she was being compared to her siblings, who she thought were just much more talented.

THERAPIST: Do you remember how we went over your suicide attempt and did a chain analysis?

TEEN: Yes.

THERAPIST: Do you remember what was the reason you gave for your attempt?

TEEN: I wanted my parents to lay off. I am not my sister. I am not going to Harvard! I wanted them to understand how difficult they are making life for me.

THERAPIST: And you tried to communicate that through a suicide attempt?

TEEN: Right.

THERAPIST: How did it work?

TEEN: Not bad at first, but now they are starting to put the pressure back on.

THERAPIST: Would you like to try to learn some other ways of communicating these thoughts to your parents?

TEEN: OK.

THERAPIST: Let's role-play. I'll be you. You be your dad.

TEEN: (*acting as her dad*) I am really concerned about your schoolwork. You are just not putting in enough time, and your grades show it.

THERAPIST: (*acting as teen*) Dad, you are worried that I am just not doing well enough. I know you want what is best for me, but I feel that you think I am capable of more than I actually am.

TEEN: (*acting as her dad*): So you are just going to give up?

THERAPIST: No, I'm not. I really want to do my best, and I want to please you. But I want you to judge me based on my ability. (*no longer acting*) So, "Dad," how was that for you?

TEEN: I started out ready for a fight, but I felt sort of . . . like I couldn't argue with someone who was agreeing with me.

THERAPIST: Did you think I was agreeing with you?

TEEN: Well, you were agreeing with my concerns, but then you were trying to get your point across.

THERAPIST: That's it! When you do that, you are making a bridge between you and the other person, and you have a much better chance that they will hear what you are trying to say.

Active Listening

Learning to listen and communicate a genuine interest in and understanding of others are additional helpful skills for many depressed teens. Listening without judging or thinking ahead about how to respond when the other person is talking is not easy. Actively listening is an essential step for the teen to become a better communicator who can effectively compromise and make agreements. It is important for the therapist to help the teen understand that listening and validating the other person's point of view will increase the chances for future problem resolution and compromise. A person who does not feel heard is not likely to be willing to negotiate. The therapist should emphasize to the teen that *listening does not equate with agreement—rather, it shows the person you are trying to understand his or her point of view.* Listening nonjudgmentally to an alternative opinion will help establish mutual respect, which can lead to enhanced communication. The therapist and teen can practice active listening in session. A helpful way to begin is by asking the teen how he or she knows that someone is "really" listening. Highlight both verbal and nonverbal cues that indicate an individual is listening. Eye contact, body language, head nodding, saying "uh-huh," not speaking over one another, asking pertinent questions, and summarizing can all be reviewed as ways of demonstrating that one is listening to the other person.

Assertiveness

Assertiveness is just one form of communication that involves a direct request. Even in the previous example, the patient had to be assertive to get her point across. However, many people will avoid expressing negative emotions, which then causes the communication to become indirect. A patient who is angry with her boyfriend may make a suicide attempt, thinking, "That will show him!" Why did this patient not express this emotion directly? Most commonly, patients are afraid that if they express their anger they will lose control, or that they will make the other person angry and the argument will escalate. So, just as with all of the other skills we are discussing in this section, we first take a cognitive approach to deal with patient concerns about what might happen if they expressed their anger directly. A particularly useful approach is to invite the patient to consider the advantages and disadvantages of making a direct request versus a more indirect approach.

The key to expressing negative emotion in such a way that others can hear it is describing the emotion rather than acting it out. The normal response to an angry person is to withdraw—which effectively short-circuits the communication. So, the way to get across to another party that you are upset, angry, or experiencing some other negative emotion as a consequence of their behavior is to state it—rather than act it out.

> THERAPIST: I want you to just let out your anger about your boyfriend at the time of your suicide attempt, and I'll play him. OK?
>
> TEEN: You sure?
>
> THERAPIST: Bring it on!
>
> TEEN: I am so tired of you hanging out with your friends instead of with me. You just treat me like dirt and I am really fed up (*rais-*

ing her voice). You make me feel like crap—why do you always do this?

THERAPIST: Why do you take all of your anger out on me? I've had enough of you!

TEEN: See! That's what happens when you are honest!

THERAPIST: Let's take a closer look at what you said and the way you said it. You said that I "always" treated you badly. Is that really true?

TEEN: No. It's just that things felt really bad right then, and it wiped out all the good times.

THERAPIST: I can understand that. But still, your boyfriend is hearing you dismiss all the nice stuff he might have done for you. What do you think his reaction to that is going to be when he hears that?

TEEN: Stop listening or leave.

THERAPIST: You got it. Can we switch places now? Let me take a try at being you and you be him.

THERAPIST: (*acting as teen*) There's something I'd like to check out with you.

TEEN: (*acting as boyfriend*) What, are you going to nag me about something again?

THERAPIST: I am going to try not to … who wants to hear that, right?

TEEN: Right.

THERAPIST: I really enjoy your company, but lately I feel like you haven't been wanting to hang out with me as much as before, and it makes me feel bad.

TEEN: Well, when you nag me, it makes me not want to be around you as much.

THERAPIST: I hear that—no one likes to be nagged, and I'm sorry. So now I'm asking you without nagging—I would really like to spend some one-on-one time with you this weekend. (*back in role*) What was that like for you?

TEEN: Well, I found myself listening to you, and at least thinking about what you said.

THERAPIST: So let's go back to our list. What are some of the things that I did?

TEEN: You made "I" statements. You reflected how he felt. You said that you were upset, but in a calm way. I don't know if I can do it like that, though.

THERAPIST: You don't think you can do as well as a therapist role-playing you in a calm situation in his office? Probably not. But I bet you can do well enough.

Improving Chances for Social Success

Sometimes, when depressed teens complain that no one likes them, it is not just a cognitive distortion, but instead is the result of some skill deficits. This can be because of grooming and hygiene, irritability, not being able to initiate and sustain a conversation, not being a good listener, and/or not being able to read people well.

Grooming and Hygiene

Sometimes teens are unpopular because of poor grooming and hygiene. The therapist can talk with the parent and also with the patient about the possible impact his or her appearance may be having on peer relationships. Sometimes, it might be effective to have a trusted relative make some suggestions to the patient about grooming, hygiene, and appearance. Some patients choose to dress in ways that push many other peers away. Surprisingly, some of these youth are then surprised that their achievement of a shocking appearance actually has social consequences.

Social Difficulties Due to Psychiatric Problems

Certain aspects of mood disorders can have an impact on peer interactions. If a depressed adolescent is also very irritable, this can be a real disincentive for other teens to interact. This problem can be managed through optimization of antidepressant treatment, emotion regulation strategies, improvement in disrupted sleep, or treatment with a mood stabilizer. Some patients who are intermittently hypomanic can be very intrusive and consequently rejected by peers. Teens with social anxiety will avoid social situations and in so doing will not be gaining developmentally appropriate practice in social skills. Youth with ADHD may engage in impulsive and inappropriate remarks and behavior due to their impulsivity. Youth with Asperger syndrome may also present with depression, but an emphasis on social skills training should be the predominant mode of treatment. Such training should be more intensive than that for youth with mood disorders and, ideally, begun at a younger age.

Initiating and Maintaining a Conversation

The skills that a person needs in initiating and maintaining a conversation include reading nonverbal cues, finding common ground, being curious about others, and active listening.

Reading nonverbal cues: People communicate not only with words but also with their bodies and tone of voice. Some of these nonverbal communications are cues as to whether they are interested in initiating or continuing a conversation. The therapist can review with the teen some common interpersonal cues. For example, cues that someone is interested in interacting include direct eye contact, smiling, interested expression, enthusiastic voice tone, and reciprocity in the conversation. Conversely, cues that he or she is not interested include avoiding eye contact, neutral or negative facial expression, bored voice tone, and failing to initiate conversation.

Finding common ground: Additionally important for initiating and maintaining a conversation is the ability to find common ground with the other person. The therapist and teen can discuss some possible themes that teens might share with one another and identify effective strategies for starting conversations. It is essential for the teen and therapist to role-play conversations during sessions and collaboratively identify any potential stumbling points. Sometimes the role play may also help the therapist and teen identify other interpersonal skills that may need to be a focus of future sessions.

Being curious about others: There is a well-known secret about having conversations—most people love to talk about themselves. Through questioning and nonverbal behavior, the person who shows an interest in what the other person is saying is much more likely to engage that person.

Active listening: The principles of active listening—making reflecting statements to show that you are listening and understand what the other person is saying, listening nonjudgmentally, and demonstrating through both verbal and nonverbal behavior that you are following the conversation—are all important elements of keeping a conversation going (see also p. 192).

Maintaining Social Supports and Connections

Therapy is time-limited. Good friendships can last a lifetime. Therefore, it is important for the therapist to develop interventions designed to enhance or establish an adaptive network of social support. For some with extant adaptive relationships, this simply means helping the teen increase his or her focus on relationships that already exist and are accessible. For many teens, friends are a very strong source of support. With emotional support and understanding from friends, it is much easier to overcome problems in living and to avoid hopeless, suicidal thoughts.

The therapist can begin by collaboratively exploring with the teen the impact that specific friends or groups of friends may be having on their mood and behavior, and to weigh the pros and cons of making any changes to their current social network. For example:

THERAPIST: Thanks for sharing your story about what happened. It sounds like you had a really tough weekend at home.

TEEN: Yeah, it was pretty bad—my mom was really mad at me most of the weekend. I guess it started with my bad midterm grades, and then we argued about how late I came home on Friday night. She was furious! She hates some of my new friends.

THERAPIST: That does sound tough. You have been feeling pretty depressed anyway, so the extra stress probably doesn't help so much. What do you think she doesn't like about your new friends?

TEEN: I don't know for sure, but she has probably heard some bad things about two of my friends who recently got caught with drugs at school.

THERAPIST: Yeah, that type of thing can certainly influence a parent's opinion. It sounds like you and your mom agree on at least one thing—how important friendships are.

TEEN: Yeah.

The therapist can then ask the teen to name his or her closest friends and circles of friends while inquiring about the "personality style" and behaviors of each. In order to illustrate the powerful effect of the teen's social circles, it may be helpful for the therapist and teen to draw circles representing the teen's social network and depict the influence of each (see Figure 7.4).

Social Circles Exercise

The people we are involved with can have a powerful effect on how we feel and what we do. For this exercise, think about your friends and family—those who are very close to you and those who are not as close to you.

In the space below, draw your circles of friends, illustrating how "big" (i.e., how meaningful and influential) each circle is to you.

Who is in each circle?

Do the circles overlap?

How do the circles compare in size?

How do you and others describe the group of friends in each circle?

What behaviors define each circle of friends (i.e., what do you do together)?

How does each circle of friends affect:

How you feel?

How you act?

FIGURE 7.4. Social circles.

THERAPIST: We get support and encouragement from our friends. That is very important, especially when we are experiencing depression. Do you think you get support from your friends?

TEEN: Yeah, they give me a lot of support.

THERAPIST: Great. Do you have friends at school too?

TEEN: Yeah, I have my old friends at school.

THERAPIST: It sounds like you have a lot of friends, so for sure you are off to a good start. Are some friends more supportive to you than others?

TEEN: I guess so. Some of my older friends don't really understand me anymore.

THERAPIST: Do you think they know how you feel?

TEEN: Probably not, although sometimes I wish they did.

THERAPIST: Yeah, I agree. Sometimes our best support comes from the friends we have known for a long time. Well then, maybe we should take a look at all your friendships, both old and new, and figure out what, if anything, could be different. Maybe we could explore how your current friendships are affecting your mood and behavior. How would does that sound?

TEEN: Yes, I am good with that.

THERAPIST: Great. Let's start with you naming your closest friends. Together, we can draw circles to illustrate your social circles and work from there.

Collaboratively, the therapist and teen can explore ways to increase contact with positive social influences. It is essential to remain collaborative and nonjudgmental during this process. The key is to guide the teen to draw independent conclusions about the impact of his or her relationships.

KEY POINTS

- CBT is based on the concept that the way we think affects the way we feel and subsequently the way we behave (and not, of course, always in that order). Socialize the teen to this basic premise.

- Once the teen understands how his or her thoughts are affecting mood and behavior, help the teen learn strategies for "rethinking" situations.

- Emphasize that the goal of "rethinking" situations is not simply to "think positively." The goal is to find alternative ways to think about situations that can help lessen the painful emotions.
- Facilitate collaboration and ask the teen for feedback throughout.
- Ask the teen to summarize the highlights of the session and collaboratively arrive at meaningful homework. Use alternative words for homework.
- Introduce *and* practice skills during sessions.

CHAPTER 8

Treatment-Resistant Depression

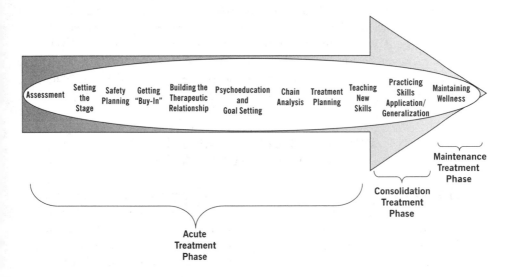

WHAT YOU WILL LEARN IN THIS CHAPTER

- Definition of treatment-resistant depression.
- Clinical significance.
- How to assess for treatment-resistant depression and identify factors that may predispose to it.
- How to target those factors to relieve treatment-resistant depression.

The treatment approaches we have discussed are the best that are currently available. However, around 40% of adolescents will not respond either to CBT or to an SSRI antidepressant. In this chapter, we discuss the steps the clinician should take in order to assess, treat, and prevent the development of treatment-resistant depression in adolescents.

WHAT IS TREATMENT-RESISTANT DEPRESSION?

We refer to depression as *treatment-resistant* if a depressed patient has not shown an adequate clinical response to at least one course of adequate treatment. We define *adequate clinical response* as showing at least a 50% decrease in depressive symptoms and a global report by the patient of improvement. Adequate treatment is evidence-based (medication, CBT, or IPT), given for adequate duration (at least 8 weeks) and adequate dose, and with good adherence on the part of the patient (see Figure 8.1).

WHY IS TREATMENT-RESISTANT DEPRESSION IMPORTANT?

The longer a depressive episode goes on, the harder it is to treat, and the longer the period needed for recovery. During an episode of depression, many patients fall behind their peers academically and socially. Therefore, rectifying this condition as soon as possible is necessary for the patient to return to an adequate developmental trajectory. Chronic depression increases the likelihood of suicidal thoughts, suicide attempts, and even completed suicide.

- Failure to respond to adequate treatment with an adequate response.
- Adequate response: ≥ 50% reduction in symptoms.
- Adequate treatment: ≥ 8 sessions CBT; ≥ 8 weeks on SSRI, at least last 4 weeks at ≥ 40 mg fluoxetine or its equivalent.

FIGURE 8.1. Definition of treatment-resistant depression.

SEVEN KEY QUESTIONS

We propose seven key questions clinicians can keep in mind when assessing treatment-resistant depression (see Figure 8.2). We review how to address each of these questions in greater detail below. The approach to assessing and treating a patient with treatment-resistant depression is similar regardless of whether the patient is new to the therapist's care or has not responded to prior treatment by the same therapist. However, the therapist will need more historical information if he or she has not seen the patient before.

How Has the Patient Responded to the Current Treatment?

Frequently, patients with dysthymic disorder or chronic major depression have not been well for so long that they may not recognize improvement, or may minimize it. It is important to track not only *how* the patient is feeling, but also *what* he or she is doing. Occasionally, parent and school reports will indicate an improvement in functioning even when the chronically depressed individual is reporting that nothing is better. Clearly, a patient who feels that he or she is not better needs additional treatment. However, there are major treatment implications when a patient has gotten better but is not well, as opposed to a patient who has truly shown no treatment response. If a patient has shown improvement but is not well, there are two possibilities. First, the patient is gradually improving with the current treatment approach, and the current treatment should be continued unchanged. Second, the patient has shown some improvement but has now reached a plateau. In this case, the treatment team may try to optimize current treatment by increasing

---

1. How has the patient responded to the current treatment?
2. Is the primary diagnosis correct?
3. Are there comorbid conditions contributing to treatment resistance?
4. Did the patient receive adequate treatment at an adequate dose?
5. Did the patient adhere to the previous treatment?
6. Are depressive symptoms related to medication withdrawal or side effects?
7. Have psychosocial stressors affected the treatment outcome?

FIGURE 8.2. Seven key questions to ask when assessing treatment-resistant depression.

the dosage of medication or intensity of psychotherapy. If optimization does not work, then the treatment team should follow the approach to treatment-resistant depression described below.

CASE EXAMPLE

A 17-year-old boy, Fred, comes in after a medication trial from his family doctor. He reports that he is "no better," and wants to stop the medication. He also reports he is not sure that therapy will work for him, either.

> THERAPIST: What was it that brought you to see your family doctor?
>
> FRED: My grades dropped and I stopped my work with the newspaper after school.
>
> THERAPIST: How long have you been on medication?
>
> FRED: About 10 weeks.
>
> THERAPIST: And is anything any different?
>
> FRED: I still do not feel that great, but my grades have come up a little. I am now able to concentrate and get my work done.
>
> THERAPIST: So when you say nothing is better, you are not talking about your grades?
>
> FRED: No, but I still don't enjoy myself much and don't feel so good about myself either.
>
> THERAPIST: If it is OK with you, I'd like to ask your mom how she thinks you are doing. (*To mother*): How do you think Fred has been doing in the last 3 months or so?
>
> MOTHER: Better. He still doesn't seem happy, but he is much less irritable, and at least he is doing his schoolwork again.

Fred's case illustrates a common pattern in symptomatic improvement—symptoms often do not respond at the same rate, but rather, some improve before others. If the therapist had exclusively focused on what the patient was feeling rather than what he was doing, the improvement in his depressive symptoms would not have been apparent. In this example, Fred has demonstrated a partial response. We would recommend that Fred not discontinue medication. In this case, the clinician could collaborate with Fred, his parents, and his physician on the next steps in his treatment. These might include the addition of psychotherapy and the possible consideration of a dose increase in the current medication. For patients with more complicated treatment histories, we find that the development of a time line that plots symptoms against treatments and life events is helpful.

Is the Primary Diagnosis Correct?

SSRI antidepressants and either CBT or IPT are the best treatments for adolescent major depression. However, these may not be optimal for certain subtypes of depression (see Figure 8.3). An adolescent patient with bipolar disorder may get worse on an antidepressant, as it may induce a mixed state or rapid cycling. Such patients require treatment with a mood stabilizer (e.g., lithium, an antipsychotic, or divalproex). These medications have some antidepressant effects and may be sufficient to treat the depressive episode. If a patient with bipolar depression does not respond to a mood stabilizer, then one can consider adding an SSRI antidepressant. Lamotrigine has been shown to be helpful in preventing recurrent depression in adults with bipolar disorder.

A second type of mood disorder that will not respond to evidence-based treatments for unipolar depression is psychotic depression. The psychotic symptoms may be quite circumscribed, so it is important for the clinician to inquire about these symptoms no matter how rational the patient appears. The treatment for psychotic depression involves a combination of an antidepressant and an antipsychotic. Psychotic depression in youth is associated with a higher risk of bipolar disorder, so the clinician should be particularly vigilant for that possibility as well.

A third type of mood disorder that may require a different type of treatment is seasonal affective disorder (SAD). Although patients with SAD may respond to antidepressants, the most specific treatment is exposure to light of a certain frequency for 30 minutes a day in the morning.

Optimal treatments for different subtypes of depression:
  Bipolar depression—mood stabilizer
  Psychotic depression—antidepressant + antipsychotic
  Seasonal affective disorder—light

FIGURE 8.3. Is the primary diagnosis correct?

Are There Comorbid Conditions Contributing to Treatment Resistance?

Other conditions either can masquerade as depression, or may complicate the treatment of depression (Table 8.1). For example, even subsyndromal alcohol or other substance use is related to poorer response to depression treatment. A patient with ADHD may have school and interpersonal problems due to inattention and impulsivity, and these ADHD-induced stressors may contribute to nonremission from depression. Sometimes patients with depression also have a comorbid anxiety disorder that comes to the fore when the depression is no longer as severe. Since part of the treatment for depression is involvement in meaningful activities, the presence of significant anxiety may block this therapeutic avenue, and, therefore, recovery. A patient with Asperger syndrome entering adolescence may become demoralized, or even depressed, because he or she may be trying to reach out to peers but is rejected and feels isolated. The focus of treatment may need to shift to social skills training, and the appropriateness of the current educational and social environment for the needs of the patient should be reassessed. A patient with complicated grief may become depressed after a loss but also experience PTSD if the patient witnessed the death or discovered the body. Treatment for these latter conditions is different from that for depres-

TABLE 8.1. Is a Comorbid Condition Interfering with the Treatment of Depression?

Comorbid disorder	Comment	Intervention
Eating disorder	Poor nutritional status can masquerade as depression	Restore nutritional status
Substance use	Even subsyndromal use may contribute to treatment resistance	Dual-diagnosis treatment
ADHD	School/ interpersonal problems may be due to impulsivity/ inattention	Stimulants/bupropion/ atomoxetine
OCD/other anxiety disorders	Interference with functioning can lead to depression; distress about symptoms and rituals	Exposure therapy, higher dose of SSRI
Complicated grief/ PTSD	Preoccupation with the deceased or with the trauma can interfere with recovery	Trauma-focused therapy
Asperger syndrome	Lack of success with peers leads to loneliness	Social skills training, emotional education

sion. Additionally, recovery from depression may not occur until these conditions are addressed. Patients with eating disorders often become depressed, either because they are thwarted in their desire to binge and purge or to restrict, or as a consequence of their nutritional status.

Patients may not respond to initial treatments for depression because of medical conditions (see Figure 8.4). First, a patient may have a chronic illness like epilepsy, diabetes, or inflammatory bowel disease that increases the risk for depression. If the disease is poorly controlled, the patient will not be able to participate in activities that are conducive to recovery. In addition, some treatments (e.g., interferon or certain anticonvulsants) can induce depression. Collaboration with the team that is managing the patient's medical condition is essential.

Another medical condition that frequently co-occurs with depression (and anxiety) is migraine. Unfortunately, treatment of migraine does not necessarily relieve depression and vice versa. However, recurrent and chronic headaches can clearly limit activity and interfere with recovery from depression. Some agents do appear to be beneficial for migraine as well as depression and anxiety, such as SNRIs (i.e., venlafaxine or duloxetine). We generally do not use SNRIs for a second-line medication. However, having one medication rather than two is much easier for everyone involved. Other agents that are used to treat migraine, such as amitriptyline, may affect blood levels of some SSRIs and vice versa. Also, some agents, such as topiramate, may have side effects that can mimic depression, such as mental clouding and weight loss.

Certain other medications may increase the likelihood of depression, such as oral contraceptives, steroids, or retinoic acid. Symptoms of

---

- Chronic illness—epilepsy, diabetes, inflammatory bowel disease
- Effect of medications— oral contraceptives, steroids, anticonvulsants, interferon, retinoic acid
- Anemia
- Mononucleosis
- Hypo/hyperthyroidism
- Nutritional: vitamin B_{12}, folate deficiency
- Migraine/fibromyalgia—consider use of SNRIs

FIGURE 8.4. Could medical comorbidity be contributing to treatment resistance?

some other conditions may present similarly to those of depression—for example, the fatigue and low motivation of iron-deficient anemia or mononucleosis. Either hypo- or hyperthyroidism can be associated with treatment resistance. Finally, some nutritional deficiencies, such as a lack of vitamin B_{12} or folate, may be associated with depression. The nonmedical clinician should refer the patient back to his or her primary care physician to rule out other medical contributors to depressive symptoms. As described in Chapter 5, sleep difficulties should be assessed and remediated, since untreated sleep problems can interfere with recovery from depression.

Did the Patient Receive Adequate Treatment at an Adequate Dose?

If the patient did not receive an adequate duration or dose of treatment, then it is premature to conclude that his or her depression is treatment resistant. Figure 8.5 provides guidelines for assessing the adequacy of psychotherapy dose and duration. Assessment of the quality of psychotherapy is more difficult, but the therapist should ask the patient to describe the structure of sessions, the main focus, and what he or she learned in treatment. Calling treatment IPT or CBT does not necessarily make it so. If a patient has attended CBT sessions but has not learned any of the techniques, then the therapist needs to determine if the patient received enough active ingredients of CBT for the treatment to be considered unsuccessful. The patient can give consent for the therapist to call the previous therapist to help make such a determination.

There are some developmental issues that make dosing of antidepressants for adolescents challenging. First, the half-lives of many antidepressants (e.g., sertraline, citalopram, and escitalopram) are much shorter for youth than they are for adults. This means that adolescents metabolize antidepressants faster than adults do and in some instances

---

- CBT or IPT, 8–16 sessions
- SSRI for at least 8–12 weeks, equivalent of 20–40 mg fluoxetine
- Sertraline 150–200 mg
- Citalopram 20–40 mg
- Escitalopram 10–20 mg
- Venlafaxine 150–225 mg

FIGURE 8.5. Did the patient receive adequate treatment at an adequate dose?

may need higher doses. Particularly if a patient has shown some response to an antidepressant, the most logical next step in someone who has not fully responded (barring side effects) is to increase the dosage. The amount of medication measured in the blood is affected both by dose and by weight. Therefore, a patient who is overweight, or who has gained weight, may need an upward dosage adjustment in order to get the antidepressant exposure necessary for an adequate response.

CASE EXAMPLE

Lori began to get depressed at about age 12. She reports that she has been depressed since then, has been on three medications, and has had psychotherapy, but "nothing has worked." A careful review shows that she received 10 mg of fluoxetine for 9 months, which was an inadequate dose. She did say that she developed akathesia at 20 mg. She was treated briefly with sertraline (50 mg), which was discontinued because she became "jittery." Since age 15, she has been treated with 150 mg of bupropion without relief. Lori's psychotherapy was supportive in nature, without any interpersonal or cognitive focus. The adjacent figure summarizes Lori's treatment history.

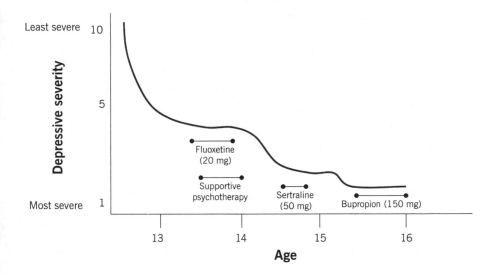

RESPONSE

Lori's depression should *not* be considered treatment-resistant. She has not been given an adequate dose of any of the three antidepressants she has received. The sertraline trial also was not of sufficient duration. Her psychotherapy was not one of the evidence-based treatments. If she is tolerating the bupropion, a first step would be to increase the dose. Also, if Lori is prescribed an SSRI in the future, it may be useful to monitor levels to see whether she is a slow metabolizer whose previous levels were too high. Finally, Lori has not had an adequate trial of an empirically supported psychotherapy, which is definitely indicated for this chronic depression.

Did the Patient Adhere to the Previous Treatment?

Treatment will not be effective if the patient did not attend sessions regularly, practice and implement skills, or take medication regularly. In addition to establishing nonadherence, it is important to understand *why* the patient was nonadherent. A patient may not implement skills because he or she feels hopeless or does not understand how to implement the skills, or because the skills did not seem relevant. The therapist should try to understand what would be considered relevant so as not to repeat the previous mistakes in treatment. A patient may not take medication because of side effects, a chaotic morning routine, or a belief that medication would not be helpful anyway. On the basis of what the therapist learns, he or she can then identify aspects of psychotherapy and/ or medication treatment that may work. The following case illustrates such a discussion:

> THERAPIST: Could you tell me a little about your previous treatment? What kinds of problems were you focusing on?
>
> TEEN: I was learning how to be more assertive.
>
> THERAPIST: That can be a useful skill. Why were you focusing on that?
>
> TEEN: Kids were making fun of me at school.
>
> THERAPIST: What were they doing?
>
> TEEN: Calling me gay, bumping into me in the halls.
>
> THERAPIST: Did this happen a lot?
>
> TEEN: All the time.
>
> THERAPIST: And what did you learn in treatment about how to be assertive?
>
> TEEN: I told kids to back off and mind their own business.
>
> THERAPIST: And then what happened?
>
> TEEN: The teasing got worse.

THERAPIST: So the assertiveness did not seem to help?

TEEN: Not at all.

THERAPIST: Would you say that this issue is pretty high on your list?

TEEN: For sure.

THERAPIST: Well, sometimes you need to experiment a little with what is the best approach. Assertiveness alone doesn't sound like it is going to be helpful for this situation. But would you be open to exploring other ways to deal with this?

In this case, the patient did need to learn how to be more assertive, but bullying at school often requires a more systemic approach. It is clear from this example why the patient stopped trying to implement the recommended skills.

Are Depressive Symptoms Related to Medication Withdrawal or Side Effects?

Patients may report intermittent experience of fatigue, flu-like symptoms, dysphoria, and anxiety. In patients treated with fluoxetine, these types of symptoms are unlikely to be due to nonadherence or withdrawal from medication because the drug is cleared so slowly from the body. However, in patients treated with drugs with shorter half-lives, the therapist should review the relationship between these symptoms and possible nonadherence. If there is a relationship, then the question to address is whether treatment with the current medication should be continued—aiming for better adherence—or whether the patient should switch to another agent.

Some of the more common side effects of antidepressants include dysphoria, mood lability, irritability, activation, increased anxiety, disinhibition, and akathisia. The most important tool for the clinician is the time line. The clinician can chart the changes in mood and other symptoms against initiation of medication and dose changes. Side effects frequently occur within 1 week of initiation or dose increase. If the patient experiences mood lability, dysphoria, activation, or disinhibition, the therapist should rule out mania and inadequately treated depression. In the case of bipolar symptoms precipitated or made worse by antidepressant treatment, the clinician should review family history and past and current history of hypomania, mixed states, and rapid cycling. If the increase in symptomatology is related to a bipolar presentation, then decreasing or stopping the antidepressant should be the first intervention. Akathisia, or restlessness and difficulty sitting still, can be extremely uncomfortable, and often the clinician must either reduce the dosage or switch medication.

Antidepressants may also affect sleep quality and energy during the day due to sleep disruption, induction of vivid dreams, or direct effects of sedation. First, the therapist should try to determine whether the sleep difficulties are simply untreated aspects of the depression. The therapist should inquire about the relationship between these symptoms and initiation of a dosage change in antidepressants to see if there is a possibility that sleep difficulties are side effects related to the medication. The prescribing physician may consider shifting the timing of the dose. One side effect of SSRIs is the induction of vivid dreams, which may not be tolerated if they are frightening and disrupt sleep. If a patient cannot sleep well, it will be difficult for him or her to achieve a full recovery. Therefore, it is important to collaborate with the prescribing physician with respect to the timing of the medication, as well as to consider switching (often patients will not experience these side effects with another SSRI). For residual fatigue in a patient who has otherwise responded to an antidepressant, some prescribing clinicians consider the addition of buproprion, an activating antidepressant. While medications such as diphenhydramine and melatonin may be helpful for difficulty falling asleep, the first line of defense after considering the side effects of medication and untreated depression is to review and target sleep hygiene (see Figure 8.6).

CASE EXAMPLE

THERAPIST: You say you feel tired during the day?

TEEN: Yes, all day.

THERAPIST: What time are you getting into bed for the night?

- In the evening, avoid caffeine and other drugs that can disrupt sleep.
- Don't engage in stimulating activities prior to sleep.
- Don't nap during the day.
- If worried or preoccupied, try to use meditation or imagery to relax.
- Don't stay in bed if you can't sleep—read or listen to relaxing music.
- Get regular exercise.

FIGURE 8.6. Sleep hygiene.

TEEN: Around 10:30.

THERAPIST: How long does it take you to fall asleep?

TEEN: About an hour and a half.

THERAPIST: What are you doing during that time?

TEEN: Listening to music. I might call a friend on my cell phone, or go on the computer.

THERAPIST: And do you then stay asleep when you do finally fall asleep?

TEEN: No, I am up and down all night

THERAPIST: OK. In the morning, you do not feel rested?

TEEN: Right.

THERAPIST: So, do you nap at all during the day?

TEEN: Yes, usually when I come home from school, I sleep from about 3:30 to 6:00.

THERAPIST: And how much caffeine will you have most days?

TEEN: I might have a coffee at night so that I can do my homework. Maybe two ...

THERAPIST: How would you relate your tiredness and difficulty falling asleep to when you started your medication?

TEEN: I had this before I started treatment, but the restlessness is worse at night.

THERAPIST: When do you take your medication?

TEEN: At night.

THERAPIST: Why?

TEEN: Because my mom works an early shift, and I tend to forget to take it in the morning.

THERAPIST: What was your sleep like when you took your medication in the morning?

TEEN: Better, I think, but still not great.

THERAPIST: And did you have this problem before you got depressed?

TEEN: No.

This example demonstrates poor sleep hygiene. The good news is that there is a great deal of room for improvement. The patient is tired because he is not sleeping well. The sleep difficulties seem to be related to depression, but taking the medication at night seems to make it worse. In addition, the patient is doing three things that interfere with optimal nighttime sleep. First, he is napping during the day. Second, he is drinking coffee at night. Third, he is engaging in activating pursuits in the evening when he may do better if he tries to settle down.

Have Psychosocial Stressors Affected the Treatment Outcome?

There are a number of psychosocial stressors that may contribute to treatment nonresponse (see Table 8.2). Even if these stressors were assessed at intake, they should be reevaluated because new circumstances can arise. Additionally, due to increased comfort in the therapeutic relationship, the patient may now be willing to disclose important information that he or she was not comfortable sharing previously.

Current parental depression interferes with the effectiveness of child treatment. Conversely, treatment of the parent seems to improve the chances of the adolescent patient making an improvement. Parents may be unwilling to either disclose or to pursue treatment at intake. However, if a patient with a depressed parent does not respond, the therapist can return to this issue and suggest that treatment for the parent may improve the child's chances for recovery.

High levels of family discord predict nonresponse and relapse, and improvement in family climate is related to improvement in depressive symptoms. Often parents and patients are unwilling to engage in family therapy. Furthermore, initiating family therapy may be premature until

TABLE 8.2. Psychosocial Stressors That Affect Treatment Outcome

Stressor	Impact	Intervention
Parental depression	Increased parent–child discord; decreased parent–child connection	Treatment for the parent's depression
History of abuse	Poorer response to CBT; PTSD; difficulty with relationships; poorer treatment attendance	Trauma-focused treatment; alternative psychotherapies
Bullying	Suicidal ideation; low self-esteem; school refusal; poor school performance	School mandated to intervene
Family discord	Predicts poor response, relapse; improvement related to response	Family therapy
Sexual orientation	Bullying, family discord, low self-image	Address secondary effects
Loss	PTSD; traumatic grief; impact on survivors	Traumatic grief treatment

there has been some improvement in depression and irritability for the child and/or parents.

Youth who are being continually exposed to traumatic experiences such as domestic violence, abuse, or bullying are not likely to recover. In the example that we described earlier, the patient was being continually harassed at school. The goal of the therapist is not to get the person to be more assertive with his tormentors, but rather to get the school to deal with the situation as is legally mandated. Similarly, when there is violence or abuse at home, either removal of the abuser from the home or removal of the child from the abusive home is warranted.

Issues of sexual orientation often contribute to lack of improvement in depressive symptoms and/or suicidal ideation. Youth whose behavior does not conform to gender norms are more likely to be targeted for bullying at school and to be rejected by their family. In addition, there is an internal struggle as the patient becomes aware of urges that make him or her different from others and open to condemnation from societal figures. It is important for the therapist to lay the groundwork for conversations about sexuality by discussing the issue with the patient in a nonjudgmental manner. Additionally, the therapist can put the issue of sexual orientation in a developmental perspective—that it is both OK and common not to be sure about sexual orientation.

A patient may not make progress in treatment of depression due to issues of loss and trauma. While children and adolescents who lose someone close to them may become depressed after the loss, a subgroup may also experience a syndrome called *traumatic grief* or *complicated grief.* Normal grief allows for a period of mourning, followed by increasing acceptance of the loss and a turning outward to return to one's expected roles and developmental trajectory. A patient with complicated grief gets "stuck" in the acute mourning phase—experiencing intense longing for the deceased, blaming others or oneself for the death, and feeling unable to move forward in life without the deceased. There are specific psychotherapeutic techniques to deal with this type of grief, and it appears, at least in adults, that treatment of depression is not sufficient. Conversely, depressed patients with complicated grief will continue to suffer from depression until the grief is resolved.

TREATMENT OF A PATIENT WHO HAS NOT RESPONDED TO A FIRST ANTIDEPRESSANT

The Treatment of SSRI-Resistant Depression in Adolescents (TORDIA) study, funded by the National Institute of Mental Health, provides some guidance on how to approach a patient who has not responded to an adequate trial with an SSRI. Assuming that all of the above-noted issues have been addressed, a patient who has not responded to a first SSRI antidepressant should be switched to a second SSRI. If he or she has not previously been treated with CBT, this should be added as well. Beyond the steps of switching to another SSRI and adding CBT there is very little research.

PREVENTION OF
TREATMENT-RESISTANT DEPRESSION

The best way to prevent treatment-resistant depression is by treating depression early and vigorously to the point where there are no residual symptoms. Without achieving sustained remission, the patient runs of the risk of developing a chronic depression, which is much more difficult to treat (see Figure 8.7).

In this chapter, we have reviewed the definition, assessment, treatment, and prevention of treatment-resistant depression in adolescents. Studies in both youth and adults show that the majority of patients eventually become symptom-free; for example, 67% of patients participating in STAR*D (a large study of adults with depression) eventually attained remission. So it is important to remain cautiously optimistic.

- Early diagnosis and treatment
- Educate—depression is a lifelong illness
- Optimize treatment
- Attend to psychosocial risk factors for nonresponse
- Augment protective factors
- Treat to remission
- Maintenance treatment—at least 6–12 months
- Relapse prevention—patient should know when, where, and how to get treatment

FIGURE 8.7. How to prevent the development of treatment-resistant depression.

KEY POINTS

- Document improvement or lack thereof.
- Establish adherence to and adequacy of treatment, including adequate exposure.
- Review primary and comorbid diagnoses.
- Assess for side effects and residual symptoms.
- Reassess psychosocial stressors.
- Ascertain hopelessness and counter with education.
- Collaboratively set clear, realistic, measurable goals.
- Be persistent!

CHAPTER 9

Getting Well and Staying Well
Consolidation and
Maintenance Treatment

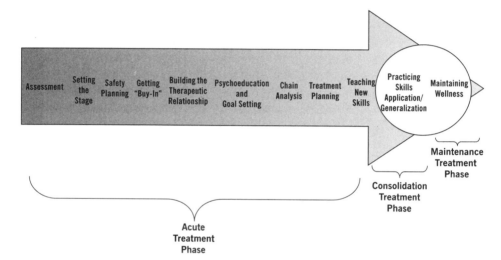

Assessment | Setting the Stage | Safety Planning | Getting "Buy-In" | Building the Therapeutic Relationship | Psychoeducation and Goal Setting | Chain Analysis | Treatment Planning | Teaching/ New Skills | Practicing Skills Application/ Generalization | Maintaining Wellness

Maintenance Treatment Phase

Consolidation Treatment Phase

Acute Treatment Phase

WHAT YOU WILL LEARN IN THIS CHAPTER

- The phases of treatment that follow acute treatment (consolidation and maintenance)—their goals, structure, and content.

- The indications and duration of consolidation and maintenance treatment for depression.

- How to teach patients to anticipate stressors and make plans for coping with them.

- What patients should look for to indicate they need to return to more active treatment.

224

■ Lifestyle choices consistent with maintenance of wellness.

■ Developmental issues in the transition to adulthood.

WHY ARE ADDITIONAL PHASES OF TREATMENT AFTER ACUTE TREATMENT NECESSARY?

During acute treatment, the patient and therapist focus on the reduction of suicidality and depressive symptoms, and the restoration of functioning. Even under ideal circumstances, by the end of acute treatment the patient is often better, but not well. Only about one-third of depressed youth who receive a combination of medication and CBT will have complete absence of depressive symptoms after 12 weeks of treatment. During the subsequent 3–6 months, the treatment focus should shift to the *consolidation* phase—so named because the focus of the patient and therapist is on consolidating treatment gains, targeting residual symptoms, and attaining full symptomatic remission. This aspect of treatment is important because patients who show improvement but still have residual symptoms are highly likely to relapse and go on to develop recurrent and chronic depression.

The next phase after consolidation treatment is *maintenance* treatment, which lasts about 6–12 months. Once the patient has achieved remission, there is still important therapeutic work to be done. Maintenance treatment aims to keep the patient depression-free and is important because depression tends to be recurrent. Sometimes, ongoing treatment for the first year or so after the achievement of remission is termed *continuation,* and *maintenance* is reserved for longer-term treatment. Because many clinicians use these terms interchangeably, for simplicity's sake, we refer to *any* treatment to prevent a recurrence as *maintenance* treatment. Adolescent patients who have had multiple depressive episodes, chronic depression, or life-threatening suicidal behavior in the context of depression, or whose recovery took more than a year, may benefit from a period of maintenance treatment longer than 6–12 months. Patients who are at increased risk for recurrence for a longer period of time may want to schedule quarterly follow-up and continue medication treatment. There are no clear guidelines for high-risk adolescents that indicate the duration of maintenance treatment, but for adults with multiple recurrences of depression, maintenance treatment was protective against recurrences for more than 3 years. These phases, time frames, and goals are summarized in Table 9.1. In this chapter, we describe structure, targets, and techniques for each of these treatment phases, as well as ways to avoid common pitfalls.

TABLE 9.1. Treatment Phases

Treatment phase	Duration (months)	Sessions per month	Goals
Acute	3	4–8	• Psychoeducation • Safety plan • Chain analysis • Case formulation • Acquire new skills • Reduce acute symptoms • Restore functioning
Consolidation	3–6	2–4	• Remission • Target residual symptoms • Target comorbid conditions • Practice skills/acquire new skills • Return to optimal developmental trajectory
Maintenance	12+	Every other month to quarterly	• Relapse prevention • Encourage medication adherence • Anticipate potential stressors • Practice skills and coping strategies

CONSOLIDATION TREATMENT

The consolidation phase of treatment involves three main foci: (1) a consolidation of the therapeutic gains; (2) achieving remission and targeting of residual symptoms and contextual problems that, if unaddressed, are likely to result in a recurrence; and (3) helping the patient return to an appropriate developmental trajectory. In this section, we address these foci and other aspects of consolidation.

A Shift in Treatment Focus to Remission

During the acute phase of treatment, the goals are to establish a therapeutic relationship, draw up a treatment contract, identify target areas for intervention, and achieve treatment response. An acceptable outcome for the acute phase of treatment is the restoration of functioning, a reduction of at least a 50% in depressive symptoms, and an absence of suicidal ideation with a plan or intent. However, as stated above, by the end of acute treatment patients are better, but not well. In the consolidation phase, the goal is to achieve *remission*—that is, complete absence of depressive symptoms.

Why Is Consolidation a Necessary Phase of Treatment?

Having depression is like being on a conveyor belt. If the patient does not keep moving forward, he or she is going to slide backwards. This is true with respect to both the attainment of full symptomatic relief, and the return to the teen's optimal developmental trajectory. Patients with residual symptoms are very likely to experience a relapse of depression or to develop chronic depression, which is much more difficult to treat than depression of shorter duration. An increased focus on a teen's developmental targets is important because in the long run, the most important therapeutic goal is to help the teen achieve an appropriate developmental trajectory. Depression, suicidal behavior, and comorbid conditions all conspire to derail normal development. During the consolidation phase of treatment, it is important to address aspects of the teen's emotional and social life that have been sidetracked due to the paralyzing effects of depression and suicidal preoccupation.

What Is the Best Structure for Consolidation Treatment?

Once a teen is not acutely symptomatic, change does not occur as rapidly. Weekly sessions may make sense if the treatment is focusing on a particularly stubborn issue, like improving sleep. However, if the treatment is focusing on increasing involvement in positive social activities, change may occur more slowly, and hence biweekly sessions may make more sense. Medication may need to be adjusted at this stage. For example, if a patient has been treated with CBT and an SSRI, but continues to complain of fatigue without difficulty sleeping, one strategy might be to add bupropion to target the fatigue; the teen could be seen biweekly at this phase of treatment to monitor the medication. Studies have shown that biweekly or monthly treatment sessions are sufficient to prevent relapse. Tapering treatment frequency also gives the teen the message that he or she is ready to be more independent. In addition, the return to an appropriate developmental trajectory is not something that occurs in a matter of days, but is a process that unfolds more slowly. As the teen begins to become reinvolved with peers and extracurricular activities, he or she may not have time to devote to weekly therapy, which is actually a sign of success! Therefore, to maintain and build on the gains that have been made during the acute phase of treatment, the frequency of sessions should taper to biweekly and then, if things are going well, to monthly. Medication should be continued at the same dose that helped the patient respond in the first place.

The Need for a New Treatment Contract

The acute phase of treatment can be both intense and exhausting. It is not uncommon for patients to want to stop treatment now that they have achieved some symptomatic relief. The therapist can set the stage for this next phase of treatment through education about the recurrent nature of depression and the importance of achieving full remission. The therapist should take care not to minimize the progress achieved thus far. In fact, the therapist should acknowledge and celebrate this progress, and then talk with the family and patient about possible additional goals, as well as the advantages and disadvantages of continuing in treatment through the consolidation phase. The patient and therapist should acknowledge the successes, identify skills and strategies that have been helpful, and target residual depression symptoms as well as other problems (e.g., comorbid disorder, family conflict, lifestyle issues) that might contribute to a less than full recovery or relapse. Finally, the therapy should revisit the patient's longer-term goals in order to determine to what extent his or her activities and energy are aligned with these goals. The following dialogue illustrates an approach to recontracting for the consolidation phase of treatment:

> THERAPIST: We have been working together for about 3 months. Where do you see yourself as far as your depression and suicidal thoughts go?
>
> TEEN: Much better! I was thinking that it is time to stop, because this is really time-consuming, and there are a lot of things that I would like to get back into.
>
> THERAPIST: You have worked really hard and have made a lot of progress. It's great that you have things you would rather do than therapy!
>
> TEEN: I am ready to go back to chorus, and also take part in the school play. Both of those take a lot of time.
>
> THERAPIST: And you enjoy them. Maybe doing those things is more therapeutic than therapy.
>
> TEEN: That's what I was thinking.
>
> THERAPIST: You know how we have talked about "black-and-white" thinking. In this case, you see yourself as either in therapy, coming once or twice a week, or out of therapy. Do you think there is a possibility of anything in between?
>
> TEEN: Like what?

THERAPIST: Like maybe meeting less frequently to make sure the stuff we've been working on is still being helpful, and seeing if there are some things we still need to address like, for example, feeling tired or not sleeping that well.

TEEN: Won't that just get better on its own?

THERAPIST: Not necessarily. I don't think it will be that hard, but it can help to actively go after those kinds of things so that you can get completely well and stay that way.

TEEN: Will you be able to schedule things so that I can do chorus and theater?

THERAPIST: Since those are really important to you, let's see if we can't find some meeting times that won't conflict. Remember, at the start of treatment, we wanted to help you get back to enjoying these activities, so it wouldn't make much sense for treatment to keep you from doing them, would it?

In this interchange, the therapist is able to explain that there will be a shift in focus and that future meetings will be less frequent. Above all, the therapist acknowledges that the goal of treatment is to get the patient back on track, and in so doing not to interfere with the other things that are meaningful to her.

Taking a Skills Inventory

At the start of the consolidation phase, then, it is important to recontract with the patient and family about treatment goals. One way to begin this process is by inviting the patient to take an inventory of the skills and coping strategies that he or she has acquired thus far in treatment. The therapist and teen can examine which problems resulted in a decline in mood and increase in suicidality, and then determine which skills the patient has been able to use effectively. The therapist should review the skills that the patient has been able to learn and use in treatment; identify likely situations in which these skills will be helpful in the future; and determine whether there are any skills that feel unwieldy or unhelpful, or need to be applied in a different context or style.

If the patient has noticed situations where he or she has had difficulty using the skills effectively, then the therapist should conduct a chain analysis with the patient to learn whether the patient experienced difficulty because the skill was not implemented correctly. It may turn out that there were other factors at play (e.g., additional vulnerabilities) or that perhaps another type of skill would have been more appropriate. Also, the therapist and patient can role-play similar situations, to test in real time whether the patient's use of the skills is appropriate and potentially effective. The following example provides a segment of a chain analysis about the patient's attempt to implement skills when faced with mood difficulties:

THERAPIST: You mentioned a time recently when you experienced a very low and irritable mood. Could you tell me about the events leading up to that?

TEEN: I was working a double shift at the restaurant, so I was really exhausted, and my boss started criticizing me and telling me I was working too slow, and I kind of exploded at her. She then told me I should finish the shift, but she was going to have to consider whether I would be able to continue to work there. I went home and felt really bad about myself. I wish I'd had better self-control in the situation.

THERAPIST: What did you do to try to cope with the situation when it was happening?

TEEN: I tried to do some relaxation exercises in my head, telling myself that I could handle this, but I was really tired and just lost control.

THERAPIST: So do you think you became irritable because you were tired and working a double shift?

TEEN: For sure.

THERAPIST: And now you are worried your boss thinks badly of you?

TEEN: She said so.

THERAPIST: Did she think badly of you when she asked you to work a double shift?

TEEN: No. In fact, up until now we have always gotten along.

THERAPIST: How long have you worked there?

TEEN: Two years.

THERAPIST: So on the basis of one shift, you are a lousy employee?

TEEN: Seems like my boss was overgeneralizing.

THERAPIST: So, it looks like we have two questions here: how to avoid getting caught up in her cognitive distortions, and how else you might have handled the situation.

TEEN: I think it's more the second of the two.

THERAPIST: OK. I don't think the problem here is that you didn't do your relaxation exercises properly. I think it was that you agreed to something that pushed you beyond your tolerance.

TEEN: I should have known that it would be too hard.

THERAPIST: Did you think so at the time?

TEEN: Yes.

THERAPIST: What kept you from saying anything?

TEEN: I did not want to be seen as someone who wouldn't pitch in.

THERAPIST: You know what I think? Maybe you actually needed a different skill here.

TEEN: Assertiveness?

THERAPIST: You got it! If you had been able to tell your boss you just couldn't do the whole shift, this might not have happened. Also, problem solving—this was the problem: You were short-staffed. Maybe there was a solution to this other than you working a double shift that was beyond what you could really do.

In this case, it is clear that the patient needed a booster session in problem solving and perspective taking. A booster session reviews the basics of the skill and sets up an experiment to practice it. In this case, the patient might start by monitoring opportunities for using problem solving. The therapist and patient can then identify a situation where the skill in question is likely to be needed and try to implement it under those conditions. In our clinic, we have a number of depressed youth who are at the consolidation phase of treatment at the same time, so we offer these sessions in a group format. In a group format, patients have the opportunity to learn from the experiences of others in the group who are also trying to get well. In either a group or an individual format, role playing can be a useful way to practice skills that the teen will need to call on to continue his or her recovery from depression and suicidality.

Anticipating Future Challenges

The therapist can also help the patient to identify situations that could prove to be stressful in the future and cause a recurrence (e.g., a move to a different school, applying to college). It will be helpful to identify the specific aspects of these events that will be stressful for the teen and outline some possible ways to cope with these difficulties. This may involve application of skills that the patient is already familiar with, or may involve the use of new skills. In any case, the therapist and patient should come up with an experiment in which the patient can test out the effectiveness of this strategy in coping with stressors that are similar to those that are anticipated to occur in the future. The patient and therapist can then role-play these scenarios. The following case example illustrates a common challenge facing patients in later adolescence.

CASE EXAMPLE

Laura is a 17-year-old senior in high school who is planning to go out of the city to attend college. She has a history of a suicide attempt, social anxiety, and depression. Her attempt was precipitated by an interpersonal conflict with a peer, and was made more likely by alcohol intoxication and sleep deprivation. Laura and her therapist identified some possible situations that might precipitate future difficulties—namely, alcohol use, sleep deprivation, and conflict with a roommate. They then discussed ways to try to avoid the first two and cope with these temptations when they arose. With regard to the issue of a roommate, the patient was encouraged to proactively find someone with whom she was likely to be compatible. On the university's social networking site, she found someone with whom she had attended camp, and arranged for them to talk and decide whether rooming together was a good idea. The therapist and patient also role-played some common domains of conflict between roommates, and discussed proactive and assertive ways of handling them.

Targeting Residual Symptoms and Problems

Sometimes patients get better, but get "stuck" with some symptoms short of complete remission. Remission is really important to attain, because people with subsyndromal symptoms are often still impaired, and they are at much higher risk for a recurrence than are people whose depression is completely remitted. Some of the most common residual symptoms are fatigue, sleep problems, and anhedonia.

The therapist can use chain analysis to try to isolate factors that are associated with the persistence of a residual symptom—or, on the other hand, anything that might diminish this symptom. At times, residual symptoms represent undertreated depression, and part of the treatment will be to increase the dosage of the antidepressant, augment it with another agent, or switch to a different antidepressant.

Fatigue

It is fairly common for patients to recover from most depressive symptoms and continue to complain about fatigue. The therapist should determine if the fatigue is persistent or is a new symptom. If it is new, then it could be related to medical issues, such as anemia, a change in sleep habits or quality, or medication. A patient is not likely to experience fatigue that is attributable to an antidepressant after having been on it for a while, but if there has been a recent dose change, it is possible that the medication could account for fatigue. The therapist should also make sure that this fatigue is not due to recreational drug use. If the fatigue is a continuation of the depressive symptoms, then an increase in the teen's current medication may be warranted to try to get complete remission. Another option is to augment with bupropion, which is a very activating antidepressant. If the problem underlying fatigue is poor sleep, then that issue should be addressed and is discussed next.

Poor Sleep

Proper management of sleep difficulties is important because it can be an important correlate and cause of treatment resistance. Assessing sleep difficulties in depressed adolescents can be challenging because subjective and objective measures of sleep do not always coincide. Still, sleep difficulties are among the most common residual symptoms of depression, and have been shown to be associated with inattention, impulsivity, depressive recurrence, and suicidality.

The therapist should first try to help the patient delineate the sleep difficulties with regard to timing and impact on functioning during the subsequent day. For example, a patient who cannot get to sleep at night and is not tired the next day should be assessed for symptoms of hypomania. Patients who have difficulty falling asleep may have residual anxiety or rumination that can be addressed by CBT. The therapist should review the teen's bedtime routine to see whether aspects of this routine are making it difficult for the patient to wind down and go to bed. Also, there may be actual sleep disorders that antedate the depressive episode, such as primary insomnia, sleep apnea, restless-legs syndrome, or narcolepsy. *Primary insomnia* is defined as difficulty getting to sleep or staying asleep that antedated the psychiatric episode. Sleep apnea is common in obese patients but can occur in patients with normal build as well. Apnea is often accompanied by snoring. Restless-legs syndrome presents with leg movements associated with sleep onset and can result in awakening or inefficient sleep. *Narcolepsy* is defined as sudden onset of daytime sleepiness.

Medication can also induce sleep problems. SSRIs can cause sleep disruption as well as vivid dreams, which themselves can disrupt sleep. Antipsychotics and, less commonly, SSRIs can induce akathisia that can interfere with sleep. Bupropion and stimulants, depending on when they are taken, can also contribute to insomnia. The patient's daytime routine is also important to review. Does he or she get enough exercise? If not, regular exercise may be of help. Does he or she nap during the day? If so, that makes falling asleep at night more difficult. Is the patient using caffeine, particularly in the afternoon and evening? Does he or she abuse cocaine or stimulants, or drink alcohol in the evening? Patients who go to bed intoxicated may go to sleep quickly but may experience early morning awakening and other disrupted sleep patterns.

If sleep hygiene and CBT techniques do not work to correct sleep difficulties, then we consider a change in pharmacological management. First, if the medication appears to be related to sleep disturbance, we will lower the dosage, see if that helps, and consider a medication switch if it does not. If the problem is mainly difficulty falling asleep, we recommend trying diphenhydramine (Benadryl, 25–50 mg) as a first step; if that does not work, we will use melatonin (3–9 mg). In girls who do not respond to either of these agents, we consider the use of trazodone (25–100 mg). However, because of trazodone's serotonergic properties, patients should be monitored closely for side effects and clinical deterioration due to the combined serotonergic effects of SSRIs and trazodone. We do not use this agent in boys because of the rare but very serious complication of priapism (prolonged and painful erection).

If psychosocial and pharmacological management does not successfully treat the patient's sleep problems, we recommend referral to a sleep clinic for an evaluation. Such an evaluation may range from taking a careful history to an overnight sleep study.

Irritability

Sometimes a depressed teen will improve symptomatically and functionally but will continue to experience irritability. As with other residual symptoms, a chain analysis is useful to try to understand its source. Sometimes irritability is secondary to sleep deprivation, in which case it is better to deal with the core issue. Sometimes irritability primarily manifests in a particular interpersonal relationship, in which case revisiting social and communication skills, problem solving, and (if family members are involved) family sessions may be indicated. However, sometimes a teen is just irritable without any apparent cause. A chain analysis will still reveal a pattern of thoughts, feelings, and behaviors associated with the irritability. Psychotherapy can then target affect regulation and distress tolerance, as well as intrusive cognitive distortions that may cause the teen to experience such irritability.

THERAPIST: Seems like you are doing really well.

TEEN: For the most part. I still am really irritable. I guess I am just a crabby person.

THERAPIST: Is it causing you problems?

TEEN: Yeah. I am getting in trouble at school for talking back to my teachers.

THERAPIST: So, is this something you would be interested in changing?

TEEN: Well, maybe we can get the stupid teachers fired and hire cooler ones, and then I wouldn't have this problem.

THERAPIST: Do you have any other option, since it may be hard to fire them?

TEEN: Not get so riled up, maybe?

THERAPIST: What is it that gets you going? Can you give me an example?

TEEN: OK. Today I was in math, and Mr. Frederickson was talking on and on about ellipses. I mean, who cares? Anyway, he called on me, and I wasn't paying attention, and he asked me to try to focus more.

THERAPIST: How did he ask you?

TEEN: He said, "I know this isn't the most fascinating material, but it would help if you could try to focus."

THERAPIST: And what did you do?

TEEN: I said that I was tired of him picking on me, slammed my books on the floor, and walked out of the room.

THERAPIST: Do you think he was picking on you?

TEEN: Of course. Everyone picks on me.

This chain analysis illustrates that one source of this patient's difficulties was her tendency to interpret interactions that are neutral as hostile, and to respond in kind. The patient's core belief was "People are not to be trusted," her assumption was "Unless I am constantly on my guard, people will take advantage of me," and her automatic thought was "Everyone picks on me." These were not beliefs that could be easily challenged and changed. The therapist and patient contracted for a second 12-week course of treatment to focus on the beliefs that were driving her interaction style, which in turn was leading to her irritability.

Anhedonia

Sometimes a patient will say that although he or she no longer experiences depressive symptoms, he or she does not feel happy. To confirm that a patient is indeed recovered, we will ask whether he or she can experience happiness or joy. If not, CBT can be used to explore the things that are getting in the way of feeling these positive emotions. Patients with partially remitted depression often continue to have anhedonia, even when many of the other depressive symptoms remit. There may be some activities that under some circumstances cause a lift in mood; it is important to identify those activities and what it is about them that leads to pleasure and enjoyment. It may also be helpful to review an activity schedule and have the patient rate the pleasure and mastery associated with each activity. Or the therapist can take a look at what the patient is doing during the week to see if there are appropriate activities for achieving pleasure and mastery.

CBT techniques can also be applied to understanding what may be getting in the way of the person's experiencing pleasure. A chain analysis can be conducted on an activity that "used to be fun," and the thoughts, feelings, and behaviors associated with that activity can be charted in order to understand what might be getting in the way. The following example illustrates this approach:

> THERAPIST: You mentioned that you have started to participate in the band again. How is that going?
>
> TEEN: So-so.
>
> THERAPIST: Meaning?
>
> TEEN: I feel like I am just going through the motions.
>
> THERAPIST: Is that different than before?
>
> TEEN: I used to enjoy being the lead trumpet player. Since my hospitalization, the band director put someone else in first chair.
>
> THERAPIST: Ouch!
>
> TEEN: Yeah, it sucks.

THERAPIST: What was it that you enjoyed before?

TEEN: People looking to me to lead the section, knowing the music well, making a good tone and helping others with their intonation, and being part of a group that sounded great.

THERAPIST: I understand that you are not the leader now, but what about the other stuff? Couldn't you still enjoy that?

TEEN: I could, if I wasn't so irritated about not being first chair.

THERAPIST: Can you try to get your chair back?

TEEN: The band leader might be open to that.

THERAPIST: OK, so we might consider that. But I wonder if there may be a lesson here even if you don't get the chair back. You really enjoyed music. It seems like a lot of the stuff that you enjoyed you can still do, no matter whether you are first chair or not.

TEEN: It just doesn't feel that way.

THERAPIST: I see. I wonder if we can try to separate out the first-chair part from the other stuff. What happened may not be fair, but I wonder if that means you can't try to enjoy what you are doing?

Other Clinical Factors Associated with Lack of Complete Remission

In our work with depressed teens, we have identified some additional challenges that can contribute to a lack of complete remission in depressed patients. These include comorbid psychiatric and medical problems, and other psychosocial circumstances. Often, when a patient is depressed and suicidal, these other issues are dwarfed by the acute depressive episode. However, as the depression recedes, the sources of these other functional and symptomatic difficulties become apparent.

Psychiatric Comorbidity

COMORBID AXIS I DISORDERS

Sometimes active symptoms of a comorbid Axis I condition can hinder remission from depression. As we have discussed in Chapter 1, we recommend that the initial assessment focus on a thorough screening for all major psychiatric conditions, as well as establishment of a time line of Axis I illness onsets. The order of onset will give the treatment team an idea of the development of the psychopathology over time that will help inform the treatment approach. For example, a depression-focused treatment is more likely to be effective for a teen presenting with depression onset at age 12 who *later* starting smoking marijuana at age 13. By contrast, a teen who has abused substances for years *prior* to the onset of the depression is most likely to benefit from a specialized substance abuse treatment program. In either case, if the substance abuse is prominent and impairing, it is unlikely that the patient will fully recover from his or her depression without concomitant substance abuse treatment.

The Axis I conditions most commonly comorbid with depression in adolescents include anxiety, ADHD, and substance use disorders. We recommend that the acute treatment for a suicidal depressed teen initially maintain a focus on the suicidality and acute depressive symptoms; comorbid Axis I conditions may be incorporated into a suicidal teen's acute treatment plan to the extent that these comorbidities contribute to the teen's suicidal risk. However, once safety has been ensured and acute depressive symptoms targeted, it may be clinically indicated to refer a teen for one of the specialized forms of CBT shown to be effective for treating these common comorbid conditions. For alcohol and substance use, this may involve referral to a dual-diagnosis program, whereas the treatment of an anxiety disorder may require targeted psychosocial treatment that combines cognitive restructuring, exposure, and either an increase in antidepressant dosage or augmentation with another antianxiety agent. Similarly, in patients with comorbid ADHD, the school/peer difficulties and impulsive decision making associated with this condition may make it less likely that the patients can completely remit, or stay well, until the ADHD is correctly diagnosed and treated with a stimulant or other agent.

The following case example involves a patient with an anxiety disorder that interfered with complete recovery from depression and suicidality.

CASE EXAMPLE

Jack, a 14-year-old in his first year of a high school for performing arts, was hospitalized because of a serious suicide attempt. He was diagnosed with major depression and social anxiety. He was treated with CBT and fluoxetine and made good progress. He continued to have difficulty with falling asleep and anhedonia, however. Although his suicidal ideation had decreased substantially, he still had episodes during which he felt very suicidal. Surprisingly, in the office, Jack appeared to be doing very well. A chain analysis of his most recent suicidal episode indicated that it had occurred at school. Specifically, when Jack had to perform in public, he experienced such distress that he decided he would rather die than be forced to perform. In the office he was not in an anxiety-provoking situation, and therefore he looked fine. His difficulty sleeping was related to continued rumination regarding his lack of social success at school, and his anhedonia was attributable to his lack of participation in social activities that in the past were fulfilling and did not precipitate such extreme anxiety. The treatment therefore shifted to focus on anxiety-related cognitions, graduated exposure, and an increase in his dose of fluoxetine. For sleep, he developed a routine of relaxation and imagery that countered his rumination and allowed him to sleep better. As a result of the graduated exposure, he was gradually able to participate in a range of activities that were meaningful to him.

TRAUMA

A past history of trauma is common among depressed adolescents, and some teens may meet criteria for PTSD. Furthermore, a history of abuse has been associated with less vigorous response to psychotherapy oriented to depression, and may require treatment that addresses issues of traumatic stress. Sometimes teens and families feel an urgency to prioritize the past trauma in treatment. Occasionally the therapist may also feel this pull. However, assuming that the abuse is not currently ongoing, we encourage therapists to first stabilize *current* problem behaviors and depressive symptoms in treatment, unless PTSD accounts for the most prominent and impairing set of symptoms. Conversely, sometimes the issues of trauma do not come to the fore until trust has been established. That being said, it is frequently very helpful for the therapist and teen to make connections between the teen's current problems and his or her past trauma history during acute treatment—for example, "Given your exposure to domestic violence between your parents when you were small, it makes sense that you are having such a difficult time knowing how to manage your emotions when you feel angry or upset with your boyfriend."

Once the teen has established and maintained safety and mood stability, the therapist and teen may revisit past trauma and discuss the extent to which it continues to affect current mood and functioning and to impede goal attainment. If the therapist and teen collaboratively determine that the trauma continues to be a central clinical concern, we recommend referral to a therapist who is skilled in specialized trauma-focused treatment.

Medical Comorbidity

We have discussed the role of medical comorbidity in the assessment of depression (Chapter 1) and in the evaluation of treatment-resistant depression (Chapter 8). Here we briefly consider medical issues that may have emerged during the course of treatment and could interfere with complete recovery. The therapist should review any change in medication, especially new prescriptions that have potential psychiatric effects, such as oral contraceptives, steroids, or anticonvulsants. Depressed youth are vulnerable to weight gain, and a dramatic increase in weight could mean that the dosage of antidepressant is no longer adequate, which in turn might account for the presence of residual symptoms. When a patient experiences chronic fatigue, the therapist should refer the patient to his or her primary care physician, who can evaluate the patient for medical causes of fatigue such as anemia, mononucleosis, nutritional deficiencies, hypothyroidism, and other chronic illnesses.

Psychosocial Circumstances

During the course of assessment and treatment of depressed, suicidal teens, multiple psychosocial circumstances may come to our attention that can have a profound impact on the mental health and well-being of our patients. Although these issues may or may not be directly linked to the acute suicidal event, several psychosocial stressors have been associated with the onset and maintenance of depression and may interfere with treatment response. As such, they should be discussed during consolidation treatment in order to promote remission and guard against recurrence. We discuss a few of these circumstances below and offer guidelines for intervention.

FAMILY CONFLICT

Conflict between parent and child not only is one of the most potent predictors of failure to achieve remission, but also precipitates recurrence. Dealing with family conflict right at the beginning of treatment can be difficult, since often one is faced with an emotional, concerned parent and an impaired child. Family sessions with multiple family members who exhibit emotion dysregulation can be disastrous. Once the acute symptomatic issues have been alleviated, the patient and parent may be able to work together more constructively. Conversely, the therapist can try to identify and enhance family factors that may protect against future depression and suicidal behavior, such as the family's spending leisure time and eating meals together, appropriate parental supervision, and enhanced parental support and warmth.

SCHOOL PROBLEMS

Depressed youth often fall behind in school as a result of decreased concentration, motivation, and/or attendance. We therefore partner with teens and their parents to work collaboratively with the school when such concerns are present. We see our role as providing education, support, and encouragement to both the school and the family. We aim to empower the teen and family to work with school administration and staff to achieve their goals and get their specific needs met. We help teens and parents advocate for reasonable accommodations, based on the specific symptom profile that is contributing to each teen's academic difficulties (e.g., sleep problems, concentration difficulties, memory impairment). Although laws vary by state, public schools are required to make reasonable accommodations based on a student's current difficulties. For example, one depressed teen who had fallen behind in school due to difficulties with concentration and motivation negotiated with the school for a "homework repayment plan": she was still required to complete the work for her courses, but was provided additional time to do so. In this way, the homework situation felt achievable rather than completely overwhelming.

Another issue that may arise in the context of school and is often related to the teen's mental health is bullying. Schools are now mandated to have policies that protect students from bullying. The therapist can advise parents that an appropriate way to begin dialogue with the school about any school-related issues is often through the school counselor. Then support from specific administrators, teachers, and other staff whose involvement and input may be helpful can be elicited via this point of contact.

PARENTAL PSYCHIATRIC DISORDER

As noted in earlier chapters, depressed teens frequently have depressed parents. Due to the genetic vulnerability to psychiatric disorders, it is imperative that therapists who treat depressed teens also screen for parental psychiatric illness. Research studies consistently indicate that current parental depression interferes with CBT response among children. Therefore, one way to help our patients is to routinely ask parents about their own emotional health. It is important to remain respectful of a parent's own confidentiality, yet at the same time acknowledge how stressful it can be to have a depressed family member. It is also important to provide basic psychoeducation about the tendency for depression and other psychiatric disorders to run in families. Although the parents frequently confirm that they have psychiatric symptoms, they are often reluctant to obtain treatment for themselves. They may report that they prefer to expend their limited time and resources toward helping their child get better. Therefore, it is important to help parents understand that getting treatment for themselves *is* part of the treatment for their child. It is helpful for therapists to have written materials and appropriate referral sources available for family members who want to pursue their own treatment. To the extent possible, coordinating treatment for a parent and child makes it easier for the parent to adhere to treatment.

Although it is ideal to be able to address the issue of parental psychiatric illness at the outset of treatment, the therapist may have more leverage as trust is established and the patient improves to some extent. At this point, the therapist can return to the depressed parent and discuss, in private, the issue of treatment, as illustrated in the following example:

THERAPIST: How do you think things have gone thus far?

PARENT: Pretty well. Jason is definitely less irritable and doing better in school. He seems more like his old self.

THERAPIST: I agree. He has really worked hard and done well. He still shows some irritability, low energy, and low motivation, though, and we could still work on that. There might be something else we can do, something that you could do.

PARENT: What?

THERAPIST: You remember we talked about you also dealing with depression. I think we will have a better chance of Jason completely recovering if you are feeling better. You still have a really big role in his life, and if you aren't feeling your best, it could affect his recovery.

PARENT: So, what should I do?

THERAPIST: I think as a family you will all do better if you can get some help, too. Would it be OK with you if we talked about some possible options?

Getting Back on Track

Whereas the main focus of acute treatment for adolescent depression is symptom reduction, the main goal of the consolidation phase is to return the patient to an appropriate developmental trajectory, as measured by the quality of interpersonal relationships and educational attainment. The converse is also true—a return to an appropriate developmental trajectory is protective against future episodes. On a practical level, while the goal of acute treatment is to reduce sadness, feelings of worthlessness, and lack of motivation, the longer-term goal for the depressed patient is to be able to experience pleasure and joy, a sense of accomplishment, and attainment of his or her goals.

During acute treatment, the patient will have identified activities that are meaningful and mood-sustaining. During consolidation treatment, it is important to identify, monitor, and help the patient enhance these activities. To protect against a recurrence of suicidal behavior, it is important not only to improve mood and emotion regulation, but also to enhance the patient's reasons for living. Therefore, the therapist and patient should take an inventory of life goals, and to talk about which ones may be most accessible and realistic. The patient can also identify which skills and coping strategies he or she can implement in order to maximize chances for success. For example, a patient who begins treatment with significant suicidal ideation, social anxiety, and depression is going to require an initial therapeutic focus on reduction in these symptoms. However, the absence of symptoms is not the same as wellness. A patient with a long-standing social anxiety disorder is likely to lack skills in developing and maintaining relationships, but these cannot be addressed until the acute anxiety is decreased. At the phase of consolidation, the therapist and teen can begin to focus on learning how to engage with peers and develop rewarding relationships. This will allow the teen to develop social support, engage in rewarding social activities that may be protective against depression, and add to his or her reasons for living. Sometimes patients cite interpersonal goals—for example, building more friendships or developing a romantic relationship. The therapist can help the patient to identify realistic and age-appropriate aims in these interpersonal domains.

Helping the teen to return to an appropriate developmental trajectory in the long run is more therapeutic than any particular technique or skill. The following example illustrates a transition to the consolidation phase of treatment:

THERAPIST: When we first met, you told me that one of your life goals was to learn how to make movies. Now that you are feeling better, is that still important to you?

TEEN: Yes.

THERAPIST: At this point, what things are getting in the way of doing that?

TEEN: I worry a lot about whether I will measure up and be able to compete with other kids with more experience.

THERAPIST: So would you say that getting more experience is an important first step?

TEEN: Yes, but I feel pushy trying to get some kind of a volunteer position, and I start thinking, "What's the use? I would just be a burden."

THERAPIST: Those sound like some of the kind of thoughts that used to lead to you feeling suicidal, don't they?

TEEN: I guess so, but this is different.

THERAPIST: How?

TEEN: Here, it isn't making me suicidal. It's just keeping me from doing what I want to do.

THERAPIST: One of the reasons you wanted to recover, though, is so you could pursue some of your life goals. If you are doing something that makes you feel fulfilled and good about yourself, that is going to be a really important step in staying well.

TEEN: True.

THERAPIST: When you are in the middle of a storm, you run for shelter, but you can't really build anything permanent. Now that our storm is over, we can begin to build something that you can be proud of living in.

TEEN: I guess I see what you are saying.

As can be seen from this example, the therapist needs to get to know the patient and his or her strengths, dreams, and goals for the future in order to tie treatment goals to the achievement of important personal goals. For example, a patient wants to graduate from high school and get into a particular college; after assessing if these goals are realistic, the therapist can help the patient identify what aspects of his or her depression and suicidality are getting in the way of achieving these goals. This focus on goals helps motivate the patient to recover, and also ensures that he or she feels regarded as an individual and not just a collection of symptoms. The achievement of major life goals, like graduating from high school or getting into college, can feel overwhelming to a depressed patient. Therefore, the therapist can help the adolescent break these down into smaller, more manageable steps. This helps the patient have a sense of accomplishment at each step and decreases the chances that he or she will become frustrated or demoralized.

CASE EXAMPLE

Betsy was a 15-year-old who had made a very serious suicide attempt by taking her mother's antidepressant medication after several stressful interactions with peers. She promised not to do this again, and therefore did not think psychotherapy was going to be useful or necessary. Our focus with her was on trying to understand how the interpersonal stressors precipitated her attempt. In so doing, we aimed to try to reduce her exposure to these stressors, reduce the intensity of her reaction to them, and increase her involvement in activities she found meaningful. Betsy confided that it had always been her dream to become an FBI agent, and she did not want to take medication because she was afraid it would jeopardize her chances. We agreed that we would avoid medication, but that this meant we would have to work hard in therapy. In therapy, we discussed what the social and academic requirements were for becoming an FBI agent. Betsy could see how her suicide attempt in reaction to social stress could be really problematic for an FBI agent, because FBI agents are probably exposed to interpersonal stress often. Furthermore, we used the idea of being an FBI agent as a metaphor for trying to investigate what was going on with her that led her to engage in this lethal attempt. Because Betsy's treatment was focused more directly on helping her to attain her life goal, and less directly on her symptoms and possible deficits, she was able to engage in treatment. In so doing, she made important strides toward the achievement of her goals.

Reasons for Living: The Importance of Meaning

It is important for patients who have considered taking their own lives to explicitly identify reasons for living and find ways to derive meaning from everyday life. While the assessment of reasons for living and their integration into acute treatment planning is important and has been addressed in the chapters on the acute phase of treatment, the therapist should return to this topic again once a teen is less symptomatic. For one thing, the patient's perspective about what is important may change with an improvement in mood. Second, it is important to continue to cultivate and review reasons for living even when the patient is not suicidal, so that if another suicidal crisis ensues, he or she can more readily access these reasons in order to counter feelings of hopelessness and suicidality.

Service activities like volunteering can be a good way for patients who have experienced a partial recovery to feel effective, useful, and needed. Also, as we discuss further below, these activities, if properly staffed, can be a venue for meeting prosocial youth and positive adult role models—both of whom can be important protective factors against depression, suicidal behavior, and other health risk behaviors. We do not recommend that patients begin these activities when they are actively symptomatic, as acute symptoms are likely to interfere with the patients' ability to meaningfully participate in the volunteer activities. For example, irritability, mood lability, and low motivation can set a patient up to have an unsuccessful volunteer experience, make it less likely that the patient will be welcomed back when he or she is feeling better, and result in the patient feeling worse about him- or herself.

The Social Ecology of Wellness

Adolescents who feel connected to their families and to their schools are much less likely to experience depression and to engage in suicidal or other health risk behaviors. Although one may dismiss this as a tautology—that is, kids with difficulties are not connected to their families *because* of their difficulties, not vice versa—in fact, connections to family members and school are protective even for adolescents with many other risk factors.

Connections to Family Members

Adolescents whose parents have high expectations about their academic performance, monitor their behavior, eat family meals together, and engage in family activities are much less likely to suffer from depression and suicidal behavior. When an adolescent is acutely depressed, it may not be the best time to try to institute these changes, but when the patient is less irritable and more able to engage in social interchange, it can be helpful for families to identify some activities that they can enjoy together.

CASE EXAMPLE

Robert was a 16-year-old who was treated for depression with CBT. One of Robert's parents' complaints was that "he never tells us anything." Once he began to recover, the therapist explored family routines and found that Robert and his parents rarely ate dinner together. Robert was the youngest of four children, and his parents admitted that when more of their children lived at home, having family dinners was accorded a higher priority. The parents had become more involved in their own careers, and Robert had always seemed very self-sufficient; he often ate dinner alone.

RESPONSE

In discussing their family routines with the therapist, Robert's parents recognized they had slipped into a pattern that left Robert alone a lot of the time. Subsequently, they rearranged their schedules to try to eat dinner together. This change in routine allowed for more natural exchanges of information. Robert felt he was important to his parents, whom he had previously regarded as "tired of being parents," and his parents in turn found that Robert was quite willing to share his experiences in school at the dinner table.

Connections to School

School can be a source of stress for many depressed and suicidal adolescents; conversely, it can be a place where healing and positive growth can take place. We have previously discussed the importance of addressing academic difficulties, problems with attendance, and bullying and other peer problems that might lead to or exacerbate depression and suicidal thoughts. However, school is more that just a source of distress. It is a place where adolescents can pursue their occupational dreams, develop new talents, make connections with teachers and peers, and participate in meaningful and fulfilling activities (e.g., athletics, performances, and volunteer work). For some patients, reconnection to school may be a resumption of their previous level of activities. For others, particularly those with chronic depression or anxiety, involvement in school activities may be a new experience and should be titrated to their abilities and motivation.

CASE EXAMPLE

Frieda was a 14-year-old girl with major depression and social anxiety who had been very socially isolated and uninvolved at school. She was a good writer, but had only been involved in this activity in solitary ways. Among her interests were journalism and work in the publishing industry.

RESPONSE

The therapist explored possible activities that Frieda might pursue as good outlets for her skills and interests. She began to work on the school paper and also on the yearbook. In treatment, the therapist worked on "experiments" that Frieda could try to test her expectations that she might be rejected due to substandard work. To her surprise, her contributions to the paper were highly valued, and she became one of its editors. The teacher who taught journalism in the school was also responsible for the student yearbook and asked Frieda if she would consider being the yearbook editor during her senior year. Her involvement in these two activities allowed her to experience connection to the school and other peers, increased her social confidence, and helped her consolidate her interest in journalism and publishing.

Prosocial Activities and Peers

In addition to extracurricular activities at school, involvement with youth groups and in volunteer activities can help to shape the teen's identity as a healthy and useful member of society. Involvement in these types of activities also tends to help the teen find a prosocial peer group. Having a positive peer group can be protective against future suicidal behavior even in the face of multiple other risk factors. Conversely, being part of a peer group that is engaging in antisocial behavior, drug and alcohol use, and depressive ruminations tends to keep the patient involved in unhealthy activities that do not facilitate recovery. These activities can also precipitate stressful life events such as legal difficulties, which may trigger depression and suicidality.

Peer groups have a large effect on well-being during adolescence. Teens with depression, antisocial behavior, and substance abuse often choose to hang out with other teens with similar proclivities. This encourages substance abuse, co-rumination (thinking dark thoughts that are shared and thus reinforced), and antisocial behavior that can lead to depressogenic life events (e.g., trouble with the law). Helping the patient to change his or her peer group may seem impossible. However, it can be achieved by inviting the patient to review his or her life goals and then noting how a particular peer group may facilitate or interfere with the attainment of those goals. Also, the patient may have chosen these friends while acutely depressed. After recovery, it is helpful for the therapist to have the patient consider how those friends were chosen and whether he or she views this group of friends differently now that the depression symptoms are gone.

CASE EXAMPLE

Adam, a 17-year-old, presented with depression, binge drinking, nonsuicidal self-injury, poor academic performance, and involvement with a peer group whose members all reportedly suffered from depression and/or attention problems. Adam participated in treatment that included CBT, stimulant medication, and an antidepressant. For the first time in his life, he found that he was able to succeed in school. He also started to consider the possibility of attending college. In therapy, Adam had identified the social context of his binge drinking, self-injury, and skipping school. Now that his symptoms were remitting, his therapist invited him to compare his current functioning to his functioning at the beginning of treatment. He was also encouraged to consider comparing himself now with others in his peer group. When asked to consider what he wanted out of life, and to what extent his involvement with this current group of friends was going to promote or interfere with his future goals, Adam was able to clearly identify how his current peer group was no longer a good fit for where he saw himself going. He continued to be in contact with some of his old friends, but avoided group activities where drinking and other antisocial behaviors were most prevalent. He took a job after school and met a new group of friends through his work. He successfully graduated from high school, continued to work, and began attending a local community college.

Intimate Relationships

One of the most important aspects of adolescent development is the ability to create and maintain intimate relationships. Depressed youth often come from families where there is a history of marital and parent–child discord. The role models for intimate relationships for depressed youth may involve abuse, denigration, exploitation, and control. Consequently, these adolescents may choose to be involved in interpersonal relationships that recapitulate these experiences. It is helpful for patients who have experienced negative relationships to identify what attracted them to such relationships, as well as what made it difficult to end an unfulfilling relationship. If a patient is currently involved in a relationship that seems unhealthy for him or her, the therapist can ask about the advantages and disadvantages of being in such a relationship. Adolescent patients can also be asked to consider what they are looking for in a relationship, and what some of the "danger signs" are that a relationship will not be good for their own mental health.

CASE EXAMPLE

Ed was a 16-year-old whose father had left the family and had little contact since he was a very young child. His mother battled depression and alcoholism, and frequently leaned on Ed for support. Ed often found himself in romantic relationships with girls who had serious mental health problems and who relied on him for help. He felt drained by these relationships, but guilty about breaking them off.

RESPONSE

As Ed's depression began to lift, an old girlfriend recontacted him and wanted to get back together. She had difficulty with depression, suicidal thoughts, self-cutting, and alcohol abuse. The relationship had been very tumultuous. Ed recognized that he liked feeling needed by her, and also that he would feel very guilty if he turned his back on her while she was having that much difficulty. The therapist asked Ed whether he wanted to consider, as one goal in therapy, how to decide if a relationship is something good to pursue or not. Ed agreed that it would be very helpful.

Lifestyle Changes That Promote Wellness

Getting Exercise and Adequate Sleep

Most chain analyses of suicidal behavior show that lifestyle issues (e.g., poor sleep or nutrition, or use of drugs or alcohol) play a role in vulnerability to emotion dysregulation. Regular exercise, aside from its benefit for cardiovascular health, also helps people have more energy, better mood, and greater ability to regulate negative emotion. Many depressed patients tend to be inactive and so need to be encouraged to start some program of exercise, despite the fact that they may not feel like it. Ironically, exercise can improve fatigue, in part because it will help to improve sleep. Furthermore, in light of the tendency for depressed patients to gain weight and to be at higher risk for cardiovascular disease, we recommend a daily routine that includes regular exercise to help these vulnerable youth reduce their risk for cardiovascular disease. Also, participation in athletics can provide positive social interaction and a sense of belonging.

As often noted earlier, poor sleep is well known as a precursor for depressive episodes and appears to specifically increase the risk for suicidal behavior. Sleep-deprived individuals are more impulsive, which in turn can lead to poor decision making. Sleep deprivation also leads to difficulty with emotion regulation (which often is already a cause of difficulty for many depressed youth) and interferes with learning and memory (key elements in academic success). Moreover, adolescents with poor sleep quality have greater tendencies to gain weight, which adds to the vulnerability to weight gain that depressed youth already have.

Modifying Health Risk Behaviors

Adolescents with depression and suicidal behavior often have other health risk behaviors, such as smoking, using drugs and alcohol, binge eating, and having unprotected sex. Early in treatment, the therapist should ascertain whether any of these behaviors are occurring. These behaviors should be targeted in treatment if they are thought to be life-threatening. Often, though, the depressive and suicidal crises eclipse these other difficulties. During the consolidation phase, the therapist should review their occurrence and discuss with the teen their possible implications for his or her life, as well as for the course of depression. If possible, the therapist and teen can work toward modifying or eliminating these behaviors. These behaviors are problematic because they compete with positive activities that can help the teen feel good about him- or herself, and increase the likelihood of a stressful life event that can in turn precipitate depression and suicidal behavior.

Patients may feel that now that they have recovered from their depression, they "deserve" to get drunk, or that substance use is no longer a risk factor for them. There is evidence that cigarette, alcohol, and drug use, even at a level below the diagnostic threshold for abuse, contributes to onset, prolongation, and recurrence of depressive episodes in vulnerable individuals. It is important to explore these health risk behaviors with adolescents and help them understand the advantages, disadvantages, and long-term life consequences of engaging in them. The therapist should work toward a commitment from the adolescent to try to abstain from or attenuate these risky behaviors.

Many of the techniques that have been described for the treatment of depression and suicidal behavior can be useful in helping teens abstain from engaging in health risk behaviors. First, the therapist can conduct a chain analysis to understand the precursors, vulnerability factors, thoughts, and emotions that led to the behavior. Second, the therapist and teen can identify ways to interrupt the chain, usually related to improved emotion regulation, problem solving, reduction in vulnerability factors, and increasing protective factors. The same factors that protect against suicidal behavior—connections to family, school, and prosocial friends—are also protective against the range of health risk behaviors.

MAINTENANCE TREATMENT

The third phase of treatment is referred to as the *maintenance* phase. By this point, a patient has achieved remission or is very close to it. This phase typically lasts for 6–12 months after the patient has achieved remission. The central goal of maintenance treatment is to prevent the return of depression. Prior to embarking on maintenance treatment, the therapist should ask the patient and family whether they anticipate anything getting in the way of their continued participation.

The Importance of Maintenance Treatment

The maintenance phase is critical because depression is a recurrent disorder. The risk of relapse or recurrence is highest within the first 4 months after the patient has gotten better, and patients who continue with medication and/or psychotherapy have lower chances of recurrence; the lowest risk for recurrence appears to be with those patients who receive both maintenance medication and psychotherapy. The risk of relapse increases with the number of previous episodes and chronicity of the disorder. Thus, for patients with multiple previous episodes, or with a difficult and/or chronic course, the treatment team should consider a longer maintenance phase after consolidation (as we describe below).

Motivating Patients to Participate in Maintenance Treatment

At the outset of treatment, patients and parents should be educated to view depression as a chronic disorder that may potentially require life long attention. This view can also be applied to suicidal ideation or behavior, particularly if suicidality has been recurrent or chronic. The most common reasons patients do not follow through with maintenance treatment include time, finances, and dislike of side effects. To address concerns about time, it may be possible that maintenance treatment can be offered closer to the patient's home. Concerns about side effects should be addressed because adolescents are reluctant to take medication that causes side effects—especially once they are feeling better. The decision about when a patient can safely be tapered from his or her medication treatment should be made in the context of what else is going on in the patient's life. We usually try to end maintenance treatment at about the same time that the school year ends, as discussed in more detail below. There are fewer guidelines about the timing of medication discontinuation for teen patients with recurrent or chronic depression, but adult guidelines suggest that long-term prophylaxis is beneficial for such patients.

Elements of Maintenance Treatment

Patients who have been treated with medication should continue at the same dose and be followed monthly; if their condition remains stable, they may then be seen quarterly. Patients who have been treated with psychotherapy are more likely to maintain their gains if they continue with monthly or bimonthly sessions. The focus of the therapy should be on anticipating possible stressors that could lead to a recurrence, practicing or enhancing skills needed to cope with these stressors, and making or maintaining lifestyle changes to sustain recovery (as discussed in connection with consolidation treatment, above). Studies indicate that patients on maintenance pharmacotherapy are more likely to stay well if they also receive CBT oriented toward maintaining wellness. In our clinic, we provide maintenance CBT in a monthly group format. We encourage the patient and family to assume an increasingly large proportion of the responsibility for the management and monitoring of the disorder by making sure that the patient can recognize whether the symptoms of depression are recurring, and how to get help if symptoms reemerge. We remain available to our patients if they need to return. If they have reached adulthood, or are living too far away for treatment in our program, then we will work with them to find a suitable referral.

Timing

To the extent possible, we aim to time the end of the maintenance phase with the end of school, so that the patient will not experience a relapse during the school year. This timing also allows us 3 months prior to the beginning of the next school year to see how he or she does off treatment. Medication should be tapered gradually, to avoid withdrawal symptoms. Fluoxetine, because it has such a long half-life (meaning that it is cleared very slowly from the body) is an exception and can be stopped without fear of the emergence of withdrawal symptoms. We usually schedule follow-up visits at 1, 2, and 4 months after discontinuation of treatment, since this window of time covers the highest risk period for a recurrence.

Sometimes the period of maintenance treatment coincides with a patient's high school graduation and transition to college. Patients and families sometimes feel that college is a fresh start, and that difficulties experienced during high school will not continue into college. Consequently, some patients may want to discontinue their medication prior to beginning college. We recommend against this, since the transition to college can be stressful. Unless there are serious side effects, we recommend continuation through the first year. After that, if the patient has remained asymptomatic, then it is reasonable to consider tapering the medication.

CASE EXAMPLE

Leroy was 18 years old, with a history of chronic depression that included a suicide attempt of high intent and lethality. He had responded very well to a combination of medication and CBT, and had been asymptomatic for a year. He was now graduating from high school and planned to attend a college several hours from home. He told his treatment team that he wanted to go off his medication over the summer prior to beginning college.

RESPONSE

The treatment team tried to convince Leroy that it would be best to continue his medication for the first year of college. However, he felt strongly that he wanted to be off medication. The family identified a provider near the college whom Leroy could see, and he promised to keep quarterly appointments. The treatment team also scheduled a follow-up appointment around the Thanksgiving holiday. Leroy reported that he was asymptomatic during the fall semester. However, during the spring semester, he began experiencing depressive symptoms again. He called us at that time for recommendations. We then referred Leroy back to his local treatment provider, who reinitiated medication; his symptoms again remitted.

Getting a patient to commit to maintenance treatment when they are feeling well requires the therapist to balance his or her role as the expert professional who knows that the odds favor continuing treatment with the adolescent's need to take an increasingly large role in his or her own healthcare decisions. In this case, we were able to strike that balance, so that Leroy was able to look for help when he felt symptomatic. This experiment convinced him of the need for maintenance medication treatment.

Monitoring Mood and Stressors

One of the skills that we teach patients and families is how to monitor mood and depressive symptoms. As patients achieve remission and become ready to make the transition to less frequent follow-up visits, it is important to review with the patient and family what they should look for that may signal a possible recurrence of depression. Typically, important early warning signs of a recurrence include a change in mood or ability to enjoy oneself that is associated with some change in functioning (e.g., grades slipping, not taking care of oneself at the usual level, becoming less social). Also, the therapist can review with the patient and family how the previous depressive episode began and what symptoms were evident at that time. For some, these symptoms were sleep difficulties; for others, irritability or social withdrawal. Every depressive episode does not begin in an identical manner, so patients should be alert to the full range of depressive symptoms and be aware that their depressive presentation may not be exactly the same in the future.

CASE EXAMPLE

Lyla was a 14-year-old girl who presented with a depressive episode that began with fatigue, irritability, and hypersomnia. She was treated with CBT and fluoxetine, and recovered fully. She was continued on fluoxetine and CBT over the next 6 months; then, during the summer, the treatment was tapered. The therapist reviewed with her the symptoms of depression and the way that her previous depressive episode began. A year later, at the beginning of the fall of her junior year, Lyla is again noting fatigue and hypersomnia but is still functioning well. What should the therapist do at this point?

RESPONSE

The first step is further assessment. Although Lyla is still functioning well, it may be harder for her to maintain the same level of functioning. The therapist should evaluate whether the fatigue and hypersomnia are present most of the time, and whether there are other associated symptoms of depression occurring at the same time. The therapist should also ensure that there are no changes in her health status that could account for these symptoms.

Upon further assessment, Lyla reports that the fatigue and hypersomnia are present nearly every day, and that it is harder to get things done than it has been for her before. She also notices some sadness and difficulty enjoying herself. Therefore, the therapist, along with the psychiatrist, reinitiates treatment to head off the development of a full-blown episode of major depression.

The circumstances and vulnerability factors that may lead to a depressive recurrence should also be collaboratively explored. These categories can include predictable stressors like examinations or starting at a new school, or other stressors such as interpersonal discord, peer rejection, or failure to achieve academic or athletic goals. The maintenance treatment plan should include achieving a lifestyle that includes abstinence from drugs and alcohol; getting regular sleep, exercise, and nutrition; and moderation in work and school activities. If stressors that have been associated with a depressed mood or suicidal ideation in the past are likely to return, then the patient and therapist can develop strategies to help the adolescent cope with these expected stressors. For example, if a patient knows that he or she is moving to a new school district, the patient and therapist can identify the aspects of that move that appear to be likely to be the most stressful, such as feeling socially disconnected. The patient can identify ways to meet people with whom he or she shares common interests, including sports, clubs, or church groups. When practical, the patient can also build contact with friends from the previous school district into his or her routine through phone contact, email, and planned visits. Sometimes unexpected stressors occur; nevertheless, the patient can review with the therapist skills he or she has learned that can help in coping with adversity.

CASE EXAMPLE

A 12-year-old boy, Ray, presented with an acute depressive episode that appeared to be triggered by a move from his neighborhood of 8 years. His depression responded to outpatient treatment with CBT. Following the remission of his depression, he received six additional CBT sessions over 6 months and was discharged from the clinic. A year later, Ray's father was transferred again, and his family needed to move out of town. His mother called the clinic to arrange a meeting with our team. We helped them to identify possible treatment resources in their new community. We also asked Ray to consider what was stressful about the move that had led to his initial depressive episode, and what he might anticipate this time around. He identified "feeling left out," "not having a best friend," and "not having anyone to talk to or eat lunch with" as the three things that were the most difficult about his previous move.

RESPONSE

We discussed ways for Ray to keep in touch with his old friends and get support from them, and at the same time identified strategies for integrating into his new community. Ray was a good athlete and had been active in his church youth group. Therefore, he was encouraged to join sports teams at his new school and to become active in a youth group at the church his family joined in his new community. We also discussed how he could talk with his mother and father, who could provide additional support and suggestions when he found himself feeling isolated and lonely. By both trying to keep up his old relationships and identify ways to make new friends that were particularly suited to his own strengths and interests, Ray was able to reconstitute a social network that was enjoyable and fulfilling.

In conclusion, the treatment of depression involves not just an acute phase of symptom reduction, but also a consolidation phase to achieve remission, and maintenance treatment to prevent recurrence of depression. Continuation of medication at the same dose that has resulted in remission is part of the latter two phases of treatment. In addition to treating any residual symptoms, the therapist should work with the patient to identify useful skills, anticipate future difficulties, adopt a healthy lifestyle, and focus on engaging in prosocial activities that are likely to help the patient return to an appropriate developmental trajectory.

KEY POINTS

- Following acute treatment, there are two additional treatment phases: consolidation and maintenance.

- To prevent the recurrence of depression, medication and/or psychotherapy should be continued for at least 6–12 months after remission is achieved.

- Medication dose should be the same as needed to achieve remission; psychotherapy can be biweekly or monthly.

- Other aspects of consolidation and maintenance treatment include involvement in activities that promote wellness, such as participating in volunteer work, sports, and other activities that provide pleasure and mastery.

- Lifestyle choices that promote wellness are also important, such as getting exercise, maintaining a regular sleep–wake schedule, and attenuating or abstaining from health risk behaviors.

- The therapist should help the teen to develop plans for coping with anticipated stressors.

- For patients who are going to college, the transition can be eased by matching the characteristics of the college to the needs of the patient, and making sure that there are adequate mental health supports available.

CHAPTER 10

Forward!

Many books begin with a "foreword." We end with a "forward," because our work is ongoing. This "forward" represents our optimistic and hopeful view that just as there have been past successes in improving the assessment and treatment of suicidal youth, so will there continue to be advances in the future. It is imperative to look ahead and see a time when clinicians can do an even better job of assessing and treating depressed and suicidal teens.

For the present and the future, the path to improving treatment outcome is to recognize that treatment must be matched to each patient's individual profile. The methods of assessment and the interventions may change, but the importance of careful assessment and a rational method for matching patients to treatments on the basis of that assessment will remain paramount.

There are now reliable methods for the assessment of depression and the identification of the clinical indicators for suicidal risk. Both psychotherapy and medication have been shown to effectively treat adolescent depression, and now we are beginning to test psychotherapeutic approaches to the reduction of suicidal risk. The adolescent suicide rate, which increased steadily from 1960 through 1990, showed a steady decline from 1995 through 2003.

Since the black-box warning from the FDA about antidepressants was issued in 2003, there has been a decline in prescriptions for antidepressants, and even in the number of adolescents diagnosed with depression. Subsequently, in the years 2004 and 2005, there was an increase in the adolescent suicide rate for the first time in more than a decade. It is impossible to say whether or not there was a relationship between the black-box warning and the increase in adolescent suicide, but regardless of the cause, this increase should remind us that we cannot be complacent in our work to help protect adolescents from suicide and suicidal behavior.

While it is true that we now have several useful approaches to the treatment of adolescent depression, it is also true that these approaches do not work for everyone. Only about 60% of depressed youth will respond to either medication or CBT after 12 weeks of treatment, and many of those who do respond remain symptomatic. Also, some youth treated with antidepressants will experience suicidal events. What are some of the approaches that will help improve this response rate and attenuate the risk for suicidal events now and in the future?

WHAT CAN WE DO NOW?

There are some clues about how to increase treatment response above 60%, achieve complete symptom remission, and reduce the risk for suicidal events. A lot of the action is likely to be in the first few weeks of treatment, for two reasons. First, the rate of symptom relief is much steeper in those who eventually remit. Second, suicidal events tend to occur very early in treatment, with the average time to such an event being around 3 weeks. Furthermore, many suicidal events occur because the patient starts with the high level of suicidal ideation and depression and stays there, so achieving a faster response rate could potentially help solve both problems. But how can we effect a faster response rate?

The rate of response for adolescent depression can be improved by using all of the tools we have currently available. The 60% response rate is based on single treatments under controlled conditions. When treating patients in clinical situations, we can look for patient and family characteristics that are likely to lead to a poorer than expected response, and can come up with ways to target those characteristics. These include many of the clinical scenarios we describe throughout this book: family conflict, parental depression, and untreated comorbidity (e.g., ADHD, drug and alcohol use). We have the tools to reduce family conflict; referral and treatment for parental depression have been shown to improve treatment response in children; and there are brief interventions that can help youth commit to abstinence from substance abuse.

OTHER APPROACHES THAT MIGHT BE AVAILABLE IN THE NEAR FUTURE

One factor that seems to predict poor response to an antidepressant is not having enough antidepressant in the blood. Low blood levels of certain antidepressants (including citalopram and fluoxetine) appear to predict poorer response, whereas higher levels predict a better response. So, when a patient does not respond to an antidepressant, it might be worth checking to see if he or she has enough antidepressant in the bloodstream—meaning that the dose should be increased, rather than just switching to another antidepressant. In depressed adults, it appears that adding an antipsychotic to an antidepressant can improve symptoms of depression and of suicidal ideation more effectively than an antidepressant alone.

NOVEL APPROACHES TO THE ASSESSMENT OF SUICIDAL RISK

Studies that look at patterns of brain activation and response to psychological probes show some unique findings in suicidal and depressed individuals. These approaches may be able to help identify who is at risk for a suicidal event or a depressive relapse, may help match patients to treatment, and may be useful in monitoring the effects of psychotherapy and may someday guide the clinician to change treatment.

Vulnerability to suicidal behavior may have its own unique neurocognitive signature and this may help to monitor suicidal risk above and beyond the patient's conscious report. Response on cognitive tests (e.g., the Implicit Association Test or IAT) could guide the direction of treatment. It may be possible to use such cognitive tests to identify and monitor suicidal risk in patients, providing an additional source of information besides interview and self-report.

Tests of decision making, such as the Iowa Gambling Task (IGT), measure a person's ability to make correct assessments of reward and risk. The person taking the test has to choose between two sets of alternatives: stacks of cards that result in low monetary reward, but lower losses, or stacks that result in higher monetary rewards but even higher losses. Adult suicide attempters who make high-lethality attempts have been shown to be more likely to choose the high-risk stacks of cards. Studies that use neuroimaging techniques to examine patterns of brain activation have found a unique signature in the brain activation patterns of suicide attempters doing the IGT.

Imagine the future, when in addition to our clinical assessment, we also administer a neurocognitive battery that measures problem solving and risk assessment—both of which are indicators of high suicidal risk. In one patient who has received psychotherapy to target such difficulties, we may see a dramatic improvement in the quality of decision making, which means that the patient is no longer in the high-risk category as defined by this particular set of tasks. On the other hand, in another patient, we may find that the same type of treatment has not resulted in improvement. This could be an additional clue to (1) continue the same treatment for longer, or (2) switch strategies. Thus the IGT, or a test like it, might be able to help therapists determine whether intervention has resulted in a change from a high-risk to a low-risk pattern of brain activation.

Neurocognitive approaches to the assessment and treatment of depression may also hold promise. Brain-imaging studies of depressed patients prior to CBT show a high response to scary or sad faces in the "emotional brain" (or the amygdala), and a low response to scary or sad faces in the "thinking brain" (or the dorsolateral prefrontal cortex and anterior cingulate). Neuroscientists believe that a problem in depression is that the emotion part is overreactive, and that the thinking part is ineffective in inhibiting the emotional brain. Those who respond to CBT seem to show high response in the emotional brain and lower activity in the thinking brain prior to treatment, and a reversal of this pattern with successful treatment. This type of approach may help us to identify those who are most likely to respond to CBT, and also to guide the length of treatment and areas of emphasis. For example, adult patients with chronic depression show a more pervasive pattern of inefficiencies in the "thinking brain," manifested by difficulty in shifting attention away from negative thoughts and feelings and accessing adaptive coping mechanisms. In preliminary work, cognitive exercises to strengthen this part of the brain have been shown to improve depression.

Pharmacogenomics examines how genetic differences are related to variability in antidepressant treatment response. This approach may help us to better match patients with medications, and also to identify new targets for drug therapy.

The treatment approach we have described in this book is about matching the different elements of treatment to the needs of each individual patient. Neurocognitive testing, neuroimaging, and pharmacogenomics may provide tools for clinicians to go beyond our current clinical measures and do an even better job of personalizing treatment for the needs of each individual.

We now conclude the way we began—with the recognition that each life is precious and each person has a special and unique role to play on this earth. Many people have heard the quotation from the Talmud we have placed at the beginning of this book, which states that a person who saves a life is considered to have saved an entire world. However, fewer are aware of the context in which this issue is discussed. The Talmud begins by noting that Adam was created as a single being, and an entire world was created for him. Since each human being is unique, it follows that there is a unique world created for him or her. The relationship is bidirectional, because the uniqueness of that individual influences the surrounding environment, creating a world made unique by that individual. Therefore, the Talmud concludes that each person, when arising in the morning, should say, "The world was created for me." This is not an expression of narcissism, but quite the opposite. It is a recognition that each of us has a task to complete and a world to build. The death of even one young person is an irreversible tear in the fabric of the world. Therefore, our task is clear: we need to help suicidal young people, who often feel that they are a burden to others, to understand that they are greatly needed, that the world will be incomplete without them, and that we need their help in shaping a world that was created just for them.

Technological advances will enhance what we do now, but it is our prediction that many of the principles articulated in this book will stand the test of time. We hope that these principles will enable clinicians to help depressed and suicidal young people to embrace the future, retreat from darkness, and choose life.

Annotated Bibliography

American Psychiatric Association. (2000). *Diagnostic and statistical manual of mental disorders* (4th ed., text rev.) Washington, DC: Author. *—At some point this will be supplanted by the DSM-V, but it is currently the "bible" for diagnostic criteria.*

Axelson, D. A., Birmaher, B., Strober, M., Gill, M. K., Valeri, S., Chiappetta, L. et al. (2006). Phenomenology of children and adolescents with bipolar spectrum disorders. *Archives of General Psychiatry, 63,* 1139–1148. *—This is the largest and most comprehensive study of the clinical picture of pediatric bipolar disorder.*

Beck, A. T. (1976). *Cognitive therapy and emotional disorders.* New York: International Universities Press.

Beck, A. T., Rush, A. J., Shaw, B. F., & Emery, G. (1979). *Cognitive therapy of depression.* New York: Guilford Press. *—This pioneering book helped usher in the "cognitive revolution" and is still the single best introduction to the practice of CBT.*

Beck, J. (1995). *Cognitive therapy: Basics and beyond.* New York: Guilford Press.

Birmaher, B., Brent, D., & Work Group on Quality Issues. (2007). Practice parameters for the assessment and treatment of children and adolescents with depressive disorders. *Journal of the American Academy of Child and Adolescent Psychiatry, 46,* 1503–1526. *—This paper, which had input from numerous experts, summarizes the American Academy of Child and Adolescent Psychiatry's position on best practice for the management of pediatric depression.*

Boergers, J., Spirito, A., & Donaldson, D. (1998). Reasons for adolescent suicide attempts: Associations with psychological functioning. *Journal of the American Academy of Child and Adolescent Psychiatry, 37*(12), 1287–1293.

Bonner, C. (2002). *Emotion regulation, interpersonal effectiveness, and distress tolerance skills for adolescents: A treatment manual* (University of Pittsburgh Medical Center, Services for Teens at Risk [STAR] Center Publications) Available at *www.starcenter.pitt.edu* and *www.drbonneronline.com.*

Borowsky, I. W., Ireland, M., & Resnick, M. D. (2001). Adolescent suicide attempts: Risks and protectors. *Pediatrics, 107,* 485–493. *—This study identifies both risk and protective factors for adolescent suicidal behavior that have strong implications for treatment.*

Brent, D. A. (1987). Correlates of the medical lethality of suicide attempts in children and adolescents. *Journal of the American Academy of Child and Adolescent Psychiatry, 26,* 87–89. *—This early study was only a chart review, but it suggested that there are different pathways to adolescent suicidal behavior. For impulsive suicide attempters, the lethality of the available method was very important, whereas for those who were more depressed, the dangerousness of the attempt was driven by their suicidal intent.*

Brent, D. A. (2001a). Firearms and suicide. *Annals of the New York Academy of Sciences, 932,* 225–240. *—A review of the relationship between gun availability and risk for suicide.*

Brent, D. A. (2001b). Assessment and treatment of the youthful suicidal patient. *Annals of the New York Academy of Sciences, 932,* 106–131.

Brent, D. A. (2002). The music I want to hear. *Journal of the American Medical Association, 287*(17), 2186.

Brent, D. A. (2007). Antidepressants and suicidality: Cause or cure? [editorial]. *American Journal of Psychiatry, 164,* 989–991. *—This editorial briefly summarizes the pros and cons of using antidepressants for the treatment of depression and the clinical significance of suicidal events.*

Brent, D. A. (2009). Effective treatments for suicidal youth: Pharmacological and psychosocial approaches. In D. Wasserman & C. Wasserman (Eds.), *Oxford textbook of suicidology and suicide prevention: A global perspective* (pp. 667–676). London: Oxford University Press. *—This is a recent review of treatment studies for suicidal youth. It is a chapter in the most comprehensive textbook on suicidology currently available.*

Brent, D. A., Baugher, M., Bridge, J., Chen, J., & Beery, L. (1999). Age- and sex-related risk factors for adolescent suicide. *Journal of the American Academy of Child and Adolescent Psychiatry, 38,* 1497–1505. *—This psychological autopsy study identifies the most salient risk factors for adolescent suicide and shows how they vary by age and gender.*

Brent, D. A., Emslie, G. J., Clarke, G. N., Wagner, K. D., Asarnow, J., Keller, M. B., et al. (2008). Switching to venlafaxine or another SSRI with or without cognitive behavioral therapy for adolescents with SSRI-resistant depression: The TORDIA randomized controlled trial. *Journal of the American Medical Association, 299,* 901–913. *—This is the largest randomized trial to address a common clinical problem: what to do when a depressed adolescent does not respond to an adequate trial with an SSRI antidepressant. There are several other papers on predictors and moderators of outcome and of adverse events and on longer-term outcome.*

Brent, D. A., Holder, D., Kolko, D., Birmaher, B., Baugher, M., Roth, C., et al. (1997). A clinical psychotherapy trial for adolescent depression comparing cognitive, family, and supportive treatments. *Archives of General Psychiatry, 54,* 877–885. *—This was one of the first clinical trials to establish the efficacy of CBT for the short-term treatment of adolescent depression. Other papers from this* *study evaluate predictors and moderators of outcome, and predictors of longer-term course.*

Brent, D. A., & Melhem, N. (2008). Familial transmission of suicidal behavior. *Psychiatric Clinics of North America, 31,* 157–177. *—This article reviews the studies that demonstrate that suicidal behavior runs in families.*

Brent, D. A., Moritz, G., Bridge, J., Perper, J., & Canobbio, R. (1996). Long-term impact of exposure to suicide: A three-year controlled follow-up. *Journal of the American Academy of Child and Adolescent Psychiatry, 35,* 646–653. *—Youth exposed to a friend's suicide are more likely to experience depression and PTSD, but not to show suicide contagion. In this paper, we speculate as to why that was the case.*

Brent, D. A., Perper, J. A., & Allman, C. J. (1987). Alcohol, firearms, and suicide among youth: Temporal trends in Allegheny County, Pennsylvania, 1960 to 1983. *Journal of the American Medical Association, 257,* 3369–3372. *—In one of our first studies, we identified alcohol use and gun availability as possibly contributing to the rise in adolescent suicide in the two decades preceding this paper.*

Brent, D. A., Perper, J. A., Goldstein, C. E., Kolko, D. J., Allan, M. J., Allman, C. J.. et al. (1988). Risk factors for adolescent suicide: A comparison of adolescent suicide victims with suicidal inpatients. *Archives of General Psychiatry, 45,* 581–588. *—This was our single most important paper. All of our work flowed from these findings, in which we identified high suicidal intent, pediatric bipolar disorder, lack of prior treatment, depression with nonaffective comorbidity, and availability of guns in the home as key risk factors for adolescents who completed suicide, as compared with living suicidal adolescents. We also identified high family loading for psychopathology and suicidal behavior as contributing to suicidal risk. All of these findings have since been replicated by our group and others.*

Brent, D. A., Perper, J., Moritz, G., Baugher, M., & Allman, C. (1993). Suicide in adolescents with no apparent psychopathology. *Journal of the American Academy of Child and Adolescent Psychiatry, 32,* 494–500. *—Youth without clear psychopathology who killed themselves were 31 times more likely to have access to a loaded gun than were normal controls.*

Brent, D. A., & Poling, K. D. (1998). *Living with depression: A survival manual for families* (University of Pittsburgh Medical Center, Services for Teens at Risk [STAR] Center Publications). Available at *www.starcenter.pitt.edu.*

Brent, D. A., & Weersing, V. R. (2008). Depressive disorders in childhood and adolescence. In M. Rutter, D. Bishop, D. Pine, S. Scott, J. Stevenson, E. Taylor, & A. Thapar (Eds.), *Rutter's child and adolescent psychiatry* (pp. 587–613). Oxford, UK: Blackwell. *—This is a fairly recent and comprehensive review of pediatric depression, encompassing epidemiology, etiology, and treatment.*

Bridge, J. A., Goldstein, T. R., & Brent, D. A. (2006). Adolescent suicide and suicidal behavior. *Journal of Child Psychology and Psychiatry, 47,* 372–394. *—This is a comprehensive review of the risk factors, course, treatment, and prevention of adolescent suicide and suicidal behavior.*

Bridge, J., Iyengar, S., Salary, C. B., Barbe, R. P., Birmaher, B., Pincus, H., et al. (2007). Clinical response and risk for reported suicidal ideation and suicide attempts in pediatric antidepressant treatment: A meta-analysis of randomized controlled trials. *Journal of the American Medical Association,*

297, 1683–1696. —*This study summarizes SSRI antidepressant trials and shows that youth are 11 times more likely to benefit from an antidepressant than to experience a suicidal event.*

Brown, G. K., Have, T. T., Henriques, G. R., Xie, S. X., Hollander, J. E., & Beck, A. T. (2005). Cognitive therapy for the prevention of suicide attempts. *Journal of the American Medical Association, 294*(5), 563–570.

Goldstein, T. R., Bridge, J. A., & Brent, D. A. (2008). Sleep and suicidal behavior in adolescents. *Journal of Consulting and Clinical Psychology, 76*, 84–91. —*These findings highlight the importance of assessing and treating sleep difficulties in youth at risk for suicide.*

Goldston, D. B., Daniel, S. S., Reboussin, D. M., Reboussin, B. A., Frazier, P. H., & Kelley, A. E. (1999). Suicide attempts among formerly hospitalized adolescents: A prospective naturalistic study of risk during the first 5 years after discharge. *Journal of the American Academy of Child and Adolescent Psychiatry, 38*, 660–671. —*This is one of the most comprehensive follow-up studies of adolescent suicide attempters.*

Goodyer, I., Dubicka, B., Wilkinson, P., Kelvin, R., Roberts, C., Breen, S., et al. (2007). Selective serotonin reuptake inhibitors (SSRIs) and routine specialist care with and without cognitive behavior therapy in adolescents with major depression: Randomised controlled trial. *British Medical Journal, 335*, 106–111. —*This is one of the major clinical trials to assess the role of combination treatment in the management of adolescent depression. It did not show an additive benefit for CBT, possibly due to the young age and severe depression of the treatment sample.*

Gould, M. S., Fisher, P., Parides, M., Flory, M., & Shaffer, D. (1996). Psychosocial risk factors of child and adolescent completed suicide. *Archives of General Psychiatry, 53*, 1155–1162. —*This is the largest psychological autopsy study of adolescent suicide and describes the role of stressors and parental psychopathology in adolescent suicide.*

Gould, M. S., Greenberg, T., Velting, D. M., & Shaffer, D. (2003). Youth suicide risk and preventative interventions: A review of the past 10 years. *Journal of the American Academy of Child and Adolescent Psychiatry, 42*, 386–405. —*This is a comprehensive review of adolescent suicidal behavior that is particularly useful in its synthesis of the extant prevention and intervention literature.*

Insel, B. J., & Gould, M. S. (2008). Impact of modeling on adolescent suicidal behavior. *Psychiatric Clinics of North America, 31*, 293–316. —*A review of the issue of suicide contagion by the group that has done definitive work on the subject.*

Klomek, A. B., Marrocco, F., Kleinman, M., Schonfeld, I. S., & Gould, M. S. (2007). Bullying, depression, and suicidality in adolescents. *Journal of the American Academy of Child and Adolescent Psychiatry, 46*, 40–49. —*One of the best studies showing an association between bullying and risk for suicidal behavior. It may be helpful in motivating schools to prevent and stop bullying.*

Lewinsohn, P. M., Rohde, P., & Seeley, J. R. (1996). Adolescent suicidal ideation and attempts: Prevalence, risk factors, and clinical implications. *Clinical Psychology: Science and Practice, 3*, 25–46. —*This is a comprehensive review of findings on adolescent suicidal behavior from a large epidemiological study.*

Lewinsohn, P. M., Rohde, P., & Seeley, J. R. (1998). Major depressive disorder in older adolescents: Prevalence, risk factors, and clinical implications. *Clinical Psychology Review, 18,* 765–794. *—This paper summarizes the extensive epidemiological and intervention work on adolescent depression conducted by this group.*

Linehan, M. M. (1993). *Cognitive-behavioral treatment of borderline personality disorder.* New York: Guilford Press.

March, J., Silva, S., Petrycki, S., Curry, J., Wells, K., Fairbank, J., et al. (2004). Fluoxetine, cognitive-behavioral therapy, and their combination for adolescents with depression: Treatment for Adolescent Depression Study (TADS) randomized controlled trial. *Journal of the American Medical Association, 292,*(7), 807–820. *—This is the landmark study on the acute treatment of adolescent depression. There are many other publications from TADS on longer-term outcome, and on predictors and moderators of treatment and of adverse events.*

Miller, A. L., Rathus, J. H., & Linehan, M. M. (2006). *Dialectical behavior therapy with suicidal adolescents.* New York: Guilford Press. *—Although our treatment approach differs from DBT, we draw from this important and innovative treatment in our assessment and treatment of suicidal behavior. This book is the single clearest exposition of the application of DBT for suicidal adolescents.*

Mufson, L., Weissman, M. M., Moreau, D., & Garfinkel, R. (1999). Efficacy of interpersonal psychotherapy for depressed adolescents. *Archives of General Psychiatry, 56,* 573–579. *—This study helped to establish IPT as an empirically supported treatment for adolescent depression.*

Posner, K., Oquendo, M. A., Gould, M., Stanley, B., & Davies, M. (2007). Columbia classification algorithm of suicide assessment (C-SASA): Classification of suicidal events in the FDA's pediatric suicidal risk analysis of antidepressants. *American Journal of Psychiatry, 164,* 1035–1043.

Resnick, M. D., Bearman, P. S., Blum, R. W., Bauman, K. E., Harris, K. M., Jones, J., et al. (1997). Protecting adolescents from harm: Findings from the National Longitudinal Study on Adolescent Health. *Journal of the American Medical Association, 278,* 823–832. *—This study shows that there are common risk and protective factors for many adolescent health risk behaviors.*

Shaffer, D., Gould, M. S., Fisher, P., Trautman, P., Moreau, D., Kleinman, M., et al. (1996). Psychiatric diagnosis in child and adolescent suicide. *Archives of General Psychiatry, 53,* 339–348. *—This study reports on psychiatric risk factors for completed suicide in adolescence.*

Stanley, B., Brown, G., Brent, D., Wells, K., Poling, K., Kennard, B., et al. (2009). Cognitive behavior therapy for suicide prevention (CBT-SP): Treatment model, feasibility and acceptability. *Journal of the American Academy of Child and Adolescent Psychiatry, 48,* 1005–1013. *—This study describes a treatment approach for adolescent suicide attempters that was based in part on our work and grew out of a collaborative effort with many other leading treatment researchers.*

Wexler, D. B. (1991). *The adolescent self: Strategies for self-management, self-soothing, and self-esteem in adolescents.* New York: Norton.

Index

269